Parkinson's Disease

PARKINSON'S DISEASE

A Complete Guide for Patients and Families

THIRD EDITION

••

William J. Weiner, M.D.

Lisa M. Shulman, M.D.

Anthony E. Lang, M.D., F.R.C.P.

THE JOHNS HOPKINS UNIVERSITY PRESS
Baltimore

NOTE TO THE READER. *This book is not meant to substitute for medical care of people with Parkinson's disease, and treatment should not be based solely on its contents. Instead, treatment must be developed in a dialogue between the individual and his or her physician. Our book has been written to help that dialogue.*

© 2001, 2002, 2007, 2013 The Johns Hopkins University Press
All rights reserved. Published 2013
Printed in the United States of America on acid-free paper
9 8 7 6 5 4 3 2 1

The Johns Hopkins University Press
2715 North Charles Street
Baltimore, Maryland 21218-4363
www.press.jhu.edu

Library of Congress Cataloging-in-Publication Data

Weiner, William J.
    Parkinson's disease : a complete guide for patients and families / William J. Weiner, M.D., Lisa M. Shulman, M.D., Anthony E. Lang, M.D., F.R.C.P. — Third edition.
        pages cm. — (A Johns Hopkins Press health book)
    Includes index.
    ISBN-13: 978-1-4214-1075-3 (hardcover : alk. paper)
    ISBN-10: 1-4214-1075-3 (hardcover : alk. paper)
    ISBN-13: 978-1-4214-1076-0 (pbk : alk. paper)
    ISBN-10: 1-4214-1076-1 (pbk : alk. paper)
    ISBN-13: 978-1-4214-1077-7 (electronic)
    ISBN-10: 1-4214-1077-x (electronic)
    1. Parkinson's disease—Popular works. I. Shulman, Lisa M. II. Lang, Anthony E. III. Title.
    RC382.W45 2013
    616.8'33—dc23   2013001929

A catalog record for this book is available from the British Library.

Illustrations on pages 6, 8, 154, 156, 194, and 249 by Jacqueline Schaffer.

Special discounts are available for bulk purchases of this book. For more information, please contact Special Sales at 410-516-6936 or specialsales@press.jhu.edu.

The Johns Hopkins University Press uses environmentally friendly book materials, including recycled text paper that is composed of at least 30 percent post-consumer waste, whenever possible.

To our dear colleague, friend, and husband—Bill Weiner, who did not live to see the publication of this third edition.

Bill's energy, enthusiasm, and commitment to improve the lives of people with Parkinson's disease was the inspiration behind this book from the first through the third edition. In his own natural style, Bill dictated the original chapters "off the cuff," just like he was sitting across from one of his many patients. One of these patients recently remembered him as "a compassionate physician who treated his patients as adults and partners in managing their illness." His wisdom, humanity, candor, and optimism will live on in this book and in our hearts.

LMS and AEL

Contents

Part IV. TREATMENT OF PARKINSON'S DISEASE

Part V. OTHER ISSUES

Preface

In the thirteen years since the first edition of this book was published, much progress has been made in the management and treatment of Parkinson's disease. There have been important developments in understanding the basic causes of Parkinson's and the role of genes and heredity in this disease, advances in the role of surgery as a treatment, and the introduction of new drugs to treat symptoms. There has also been increased interest in research on disease-modifying or neuroprotective therapies that may slow the progression of Parkinson's. This new edition discusses all of these developments and retains the original intent and purpose of the book to help patients and their families develop a fuller understanding of what living with Parkinson's disease is like. When people first learn of the diagnosis of Parkinson's disease, they generally know little about this illness. Understandably, a myriad of questions arise. Many patients and families become alarmed as they translate their limited experience and knowledge to themselves. The fact is that the effect of Parkinson's disease on people's lives has been fundamentally altered in recent years, as new and better treatments have become available.

Indeed, Parkinson's disease has become a disorder that does not prevent people from living productive and satisfying lives for many years. In fact, a large proportion of those with Parkinson's disease remain independent in the activities of daily living (ADL) ten years after diagnosis. Understanding the symptoms of Parkinson's disease and the management of the disease is the key to each person's ability to preserve his or her sense of stability and control. There are many examples of medical conditions that are chronic illnesses, including arthritis, asthma, diabetes, and Parkinson's disease. In every one of these examples, the recipe for living well with the disorder involves having a clear understanding of both the medical condition and the pivotal role that a prepared individual can assume in the management of his or her own health. For example, in making clinical decisions, a physician relies on the history and feedback that the patient and caregivers provide. There is no one formula for the successful management of Parkinson's disease. Instead, success relies upon an individualized and comprehensive plan of care based on shared decision-making between the experienced physician and the prepared patient.

We have written a book that explores Parkinson's disease in straightforward and honest terms. We have explained what goes wrong in the brain that leads to the disorder, and we have also explained how a physician goes about making the diagnosis of Parkinson's disease. We have discussed the subtleties involved in diagnosis, so people with Parkinson's disease and their families understand the challenges that sometimes arise in arriving at a correct diagnosis.

Parkinson's disease is a progressive problem that gradually worsens with time. In separate chapters we have delineated the common problems associated with the early, middle, and advanced stages of Parkinson's disease. We not only discuss these problems in considerable detail but also offer numerous suggestions based on our experiences regarding how to better live with these problems.

Most people think that the major problems of Parkinson's disease relate to problems with movement, including tremor and walking. However, patients with many years of experience with Parkinson's are also familiar with a wide array of nonmotor symptoms, both due to the disease and its treatment. Therefore, we have a separate chapter (Chapter 6) in which we extensively review the common nonmotor symptoms that may occur, including depression, apathy, anxiety, sweating, sexual dysfunction, memory problems, sleep disturbance, impulse control disorders (for example, excessive gambling, shopping, computer use, eating), bladder problems, and constipation.

The role of drug therapy in the treatment of Parkinson's disease is thoroughly discussed in this book. In the last forty-five years, impressive advances in the therapy of Parkinson's disease have been made. We outline how Parkinson's drugs work, why they are helpful, the side effects associated with them, and what patients can realistically expect of each of them. How to use medications safely and effectively, and the various drug combinations, are also thoroughly reviewed, as is drug therapy for the various nonmotor symptoms.

The role of surgery in the treatment of Parkinson's disease continues to evolve. We review the different types of surgery that can be of value in Parkinson's disease. Importantly, we present the key questions that patients and families should ask themselves and their physician before considering surgery as a therapeutic option.

The book closes with a long chapter of commonly asked questions and clear and concise answers to these many difficult questions that often arise during an office visit. (The subject of each question and answer is covered in much greater detail in the many chapters within the book.)

Our many years of experience with taking care of patients with Parkinson's disease have taught us that well-informed, knowledgeable patients do better over time. Our goal in this edition is to contribute to a foundation of knowledge for persons who are living with Parkinson's disease in order to help them make healthy adjustments to these changes, to develop competency in self-monitoring and self-management, and to become effective partners in shared decision-making with their physician. The chapters of the book can be read in sequence, but they can also be read separately. To permit this approach, we have incorporated a certain amount of duplication in the information provided. For those reading chapters in sequence, this can serve to reinforce the important issues covered.

We thank all the patients and families whom we have taken care of over the years, for sharing with us their insights, experiences, and responses to Parkinson's disease. The spirit that the Parkinson's community exhibits is an enduring inspiration. We hope that we successfully communicate the world conveyed by our patients to the larger community of persons and families affected by Parkinson's disease.

We thank Cheryl Grant-Johnson and Cherika Greene, who have diligently supported us with fine administrative skills during the preparation of this book. We thank our editors, Jacqueline Wehmueller of the Johns Hopkins University Press as well as Alice Lium and Linda Strange, who helped us transform our initial text into an easily readable and patient-friendly format. We also thank special benefactors who have generously supported our research on this project as well as many other Parkinson's disease–related projects: Rosalyn Newman, Morton Shulman, Jack and Mary Clark, the Catherine Manson family, Lily Safra and the Edmond J. Safra Philanthropic Foundation, the Eugenia Brin family, and the Frederick Henry Prince Trust.

Part I

INTRODUCTION

CHAPTER I

What Is
Parkinson's Disease?

- *What are the symptoms of Parkinson's disease?*
- *What causes these symptoms?*
- *What is the difference between Parkinson's disease and parkinsonism?*
- *When should I tell people that I have Parkinson's?*

Whenever a diagnosis of Parkinson's disease is made, patients and families naturally ask, "What *is* Parkinson's disease?" As doctors treating people who have Parkinson's, of course, we discuss this question with many patients. But we—and they—are aware that the answer is both straightforward and elusive.

Parkinson's disease is a degenerative neurologic disease. *Degenerative* means "declining in quality"—thus, the disease increases in severity over time; *neurologic* refers to the nervous system. One could therefore say that Parkinson's disease is a disease of the nervous system that gets worse over time.

We also describe Parkinson's disease as a chronic, progressive neurologic disease. *Chronic* means "of long duration"; *progressive* means "proceeding in steps" or "advancing." Parkinson's disease does not go away, and it gradually gets worse.

Parkinson's disease is named after the English physician James Parkinson, who first described the illness. His original paper describing this disorder, published in 1817, was titled "Essay on the Shaking Palsy," and to this day Parkinson's disease is still sometimes called the "shaking palsy." Ancient medical writings include descriptions of people with a disorder that fits the clinical picture of this disease, but Parkinson is given credit for providing the most thorough description of it. Another name for this illness is *paralysis agitans*, which is simply the Latin translation of "shaking palsy." The names *Parkinson's disease, shaking palsy,* and *paralysis agitans* all refer to the same illness.

There is some good news. True Parkinson's disease progresses slowly. Even after the symptoms have become clear enough to allow a definitive diagnosis, it is usually years, maybe ten or more years, before a person suffers from a serious disability. Further, treatments are available that relieve symptoms, so that years, sometimes a decade or more, can go by before symptoms have a significant impact on a person's quality of life.

In people who have Parkinson's disease, specific groups of brain cells called *neurons* are slowly and progressively injured, then selectively degenerate or die. This process causes the typical symptoms of Parkinson's disease, which doctors call "characteristic symptoms" because they are the major features of Parkinson's. (In this book, when we say symptoms are "characteristic" of or "characterize" a disorder, we mean they are typical of that particular disorder and distinguish it from others.)

These are the characteristic symptoms of Parkinson's disease: People who have Parkinson's may tremble involuntarily. They find their muscles become rigid and stiff, and they lose their ability to make rapid, spontaneous movements. They walk in a recognizable manner, with a typical gait in which the body is bent or flexed, and they may have difficulty maintaining their balance. These symptoms do not emerge all at once. For example, walking may become slower and may not worsen for years. Balance is unlikely to be a problem until the more advanced stages. And tremor, the most recognizable feature, does not occur in everyone. The characteristic symptoms of moderate Parkinson's disease can be remembered with the acronym TRAP: *T* is for *tremor* and *R* for *rigidity*. *A* is for *akinesia* (meaning, literally, "lack of movement"), referring to the loss of spontaneous or voluntary movement and loss of fluid motion (the slowing down, rather than complete loss, of movement is called *bradykinesia*). *P* is for *postural instability,* which involves

TABLE I.I

CHARACTERISTIC SIGNS AND SYMPTOMS OF PARKINSON'S DISEASE

T	Tremor	Involuntary trembling of the limbs (often the initial symptom)
R	Rigidity	Stiffness of the muscles
A	Akinesia	Lack of movement or slowness in initiating and maintaining movement
P	Postural instability	Characteristic bending or flexion of the body, associated with difficulty in maintaining balance and disturbances in gait

difficulties with balance and the risk of falling (Table 1.1). Parkinson's has neither a cure nor any treatment to slow down its progression.

Furthermore, the signs and symptoms* of early Parkinson's are only subtly different from those of other neurologic diseases, some more serious and some less serious than Parkinson's. The similarities among these diseases can make diagnosis difficult, and as frustrating as it may be for a person who has Parkinson's symptoms, often the only way to identify Parkinson's disease for sure is to wait and see (see Chapter 8).

WHAT HAPPENS IN PARKINSON'S DISEASE?

In Parkinson's disease, neurons (nerve cells) of the brain area known as the *substantia nigra* (Latin for "black substance") are primarily affected (Figure 1.1). When neurons in the substantia nigra degenerate, the brain's ability to generate body movements is disrupted, and this disruption produces signs and symptoms characteristic of Parkinson's disease—tremor; rigidity; akinesia (lack of movement or loss of spontaneous movement) and bradykinesia (slowness of movement); and problems with walking and posture. Other areas of the brain are also affected, especially later in the disease, and it is this aspect of the dis-

---

Symptoms are what the patient complains of; *signs* are what the doctor finds on examination. Parkinson's has both signs and symptoms that are typical of the disease. We discuss them in depth in later chapters.

FIGURE 1.1 Location of the substantia nigra (the area of the brain that contains dopamine cells), deep within the brain. The large cerebral hemispheres enclose and cover the substantia nigra as well as other deep midbrain structures.

ease that likely accounts for the broad spectrum of symptoms that can eventually be a part of the illness.

The symptoms of any brain disease are determined in part by the location of the neurons that degenerate. For example, Alzheimer's disease involves the degeneration of neurons of the cerebral cortex and results in memory loss and mental deterioration. In amyotrophic lateral sclerosis (ALS, or Lou Gehrig's disease), the selective death of motor neurons in the spinal cord and brain causes profound motor weakness. Again, in Parkinson's disease, the affected neurons are especially those located in the substantia nigra, an area of the brain that is important for control and regulation of motor activity (movement).

WHAT CAUSES THE SYMPTOMS?

The substantia nigra is a very small area located deep within the brain. There is one substantia nigra on the right side of the brain and one on the left, but for ease of discussion, the medical literature refers to them as if they were a single structure. The symptoms of Parkinson's disease do not become noticeable until about 50 to 70 percent of the cells of the substantia nigra have died, because the human nervous system has multiple safety factors and redundancies built into it. For a long time, these safety factors are able to take over the activities of the dying cells.

In autopsies of persons who had Parkinson's disease, the brain appears to be relatively normal except that the substantia nigra has lost its usual black pigment (Figure 1.2). Under the microscope we can see substantially fewer cells in this substantia nigra than in that of healthy brains, and the remaining cells often show signs of abnormality. One hallmark of Parkinson's disease is the presence of small bodies known as *Lewy bodies* within the remaining substantia nigra cells.

The substantia nigra accounts for an extremely small percentage of the brain's weight, but because of its important electrochemical connections with motor centers (brain centers that control movement), it is a vital component in how we move. Specifically, a series of complicated electrical and chemical events within the brain transmits information from neuron to neuron. The chemicals that brain cells use to commu-

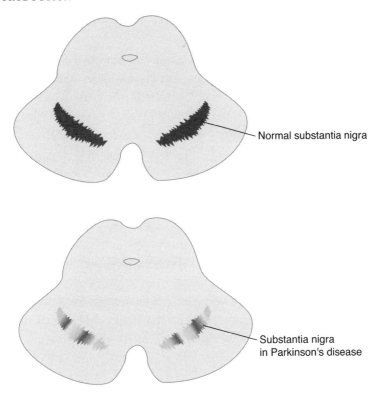

FIGURE 1.2 The *top panel* shows the normal substantia nigra with its dark pigment that gives it the characteristic black color. This is the actual appearance that is seen by the naked eye when this part of the brain is examined. The *bottom panel* with the faded pale area in the region of the substantia nigra is the characteristic finding seen with the naked eye in the brain of a patient with Parkinson's disease. The loss of the dopamine-containing pigmented black cells within the substantia nigra is the landmark pathologic feature of Parkinson's disease.

nicate with one another are called *neurotransmitters* or, more generally, *neurochemicals*. The specific neurotransmitter produced and used by the substantia nigra is *dopamine*. When the cells of the substantia nigra degenerate and die, dopamine is lost and dopamine-relayed messages to other motor centers cannot go through. This is the primary cause of most of the motor symptoms in Parkinson's disease.

Recent technological advances in imaging techniques allow visualization of the dopaminergic cells in the substantia nigra in the living brain (Figure 1.3). Several different types of imaging can be used, including positron emission tomography (PET) or single photon emission computerized tomography (SPECT). These techniques combine biology, pharmacology, computerized systems, and special laboratories to make radio pharmaceuticals that can be injected in patients and seen during imaging. One test that is now available is SPECT. A particular type of SPECT Scan is the DATScan. Although this test can distinguish normal from abnormal dopamine pathways, whether or not it will be helpful in diagnosis remains to be seen. We will discuss the advantages and disadvantages of this test in Chapter 8.

There is more. While the loss of dopamine-producing cells is the primary neurochemical disturbance in Parkinson's, the neurochemical disturbances are not limited to the cells of the substantia nigra and to the loss of dopamine. Other small nuclear centers within the brain

FIGURE 1.3 Positron Emission Tomography (PET) scan using the ligand [¹¹C] dihydrotetrabenazine (DBTZ) (*light-colored regions*) superimposed on brain MRIs. This shows dopamine storage in the terminals of dopamine neurons in the striatum (*thicker arrows; left*). In Parkinson's disease there is a loss of these terminals, especially in the putamen. Note the tails on the comma-shaped regions in the normal scan (*thinner arrows*) and the loss of these tails in the Parkinson's scan (*right*). Courtesy of Dr. A. Strafella.

(e.g., the regions called the *dorsal motor nucleus of the vagus* and the *locus ceruleus*) also are affected by the degeneration. In Parkinson's disease, as the concentrations of dopamine in the brain decline, so do concentrations of other neurotransmitters such as norepinephrine and serotonin, although changes in these other neurotransmitters are not nearly as significant as the loss of dopamine. These neurotransmitter and cell changes are spread widely throughout the brain, which may help explain why dopamine replacement does not correct all the problems caused by Parkinson's. For example, dopamine replacement is very helpful for slowness (bradykinesia) and rigidity but generally is not helpful for balance. In short, Parkinson's disease is not just a dopamine deficiency state.

Although we have some understanding that neurochemical disturbance causes the symptoms of Parkinson's, we still do not know what causes the neurodegeneration, although extensive scientific research has been conducted in this area. For this reason, the disease is sometimes termed *idiopathic* (cause unknown) Parkinson's disease. In Chapter 2 we look at what the current research indicates, and in Chapter 18 we investigate some leads that may shed light on the causes.

Because the brain's neurotransmitters—especially dopamine—are so important to the central nervous system's control of the muscles, when these neurotransmitters are in short supply, the muscles act strangely. The central mechanism that controls muscle tone is altered. The muscles may tighten up at inappropriate times—rapid tightening and releasing of muscles produces a tremor. Sometimes the muscles tighten up and become stiff and rigid. With inadequate communication between the brain and the muscles, movement also becomes slow: muscles cannot make quick, fluid, spontaneous movements. The central mechanism that controls muscle tone does not function adequately for the delicate interplay of muscles required to help us stand, walk, and balance. In addition, because Parkinson's disease also affects the autonomic nervous system (the largely unconscious system that controls our body temperature, digestive system, sexual function, and bladder control, among other functions), these systems may also act oddly.

In true Parkinson's disease, the first symptoms differ only slightly from the normal state and progress slowly, perhaps over decades. Different people have different combinations of symptoms.

PARKINSONISM

Any person who has the signs and symptoms characteristic of Parkinson's disease (tremor, rigidity, slowness of movement or loss of spontaneous movement, and postural impairment) is said to have *parkinsonism,* but not every person who has parkinsonism has Parkinson's disease. Parkinsonism has many possible causes, and Parkinson's disease is only one of the possibilities. For example, parkinsonism may be the result of a stroke or a side effect of certain medications. Many other types of neurodegenerative disorders result in parkinsonism, although Parkinson's disease is the most common of these. In many cases the parkinsonism found in these other disorders is due to damage to the substantia nigra, and more often than not the damage extends to other brain areas as well. People who have parkinsonism may have symptoms of impaired movement, thinking, behavior, and other body functions (such as blood pressure and sexual, bladder, and bowel function) that people who have true Parkinson's are less likely to develop.

Even considering such differences, Parkinson's disease can be very difficult to distinguish from other forms of parkinsonism. Patients and their families need to understand parkinsonism, because some 20 to 25 percent of people diagnosed with Parkinson's disease will eventually be discovered to have some other form of parkinsonism. Parkinsonism may look like Parkinson's disease, but over time it does not act like it. Differences that were subtle at the beginning of a disorder often become more pronounced as it progresses. For people who have parkinsonism, the symptoms may become more disabling more quickly or may progress more slowly than in Parkinson's disease. Parkinsonism symptoms may or may not respond to the medications used to treat Parkinson's disease.

A number of other disorders that include involuntary tremor are not, strictly speaking, a type of parkinsonism but can also be mistaken for Parkinson's disease.

TABLE 1.2

DISEASES THAT CAN BE MISTAKEN FOR PARKINSON'S DISEASE

Disease	Signs, Symptoms, and Features That Distinguish It from Parkinson's
Progressive supranuclear palsy (PSP)	Parkinsonism plus early falling and difficulty moving the eyes
Multiple system atrophy (MSA) Shy-Drager syndrome Striatonigral degeneration Olivopontocerebellar degeneration	Parkinsonism plus blood pressure regulation problems (dizziness and fainting on standing), urinary problems (frequency, urgency), sexual dysfunction, poor response to antiparkinson medications
Multiple small strokes	No clear history of sudden stroke; affects legs more than arms; not much tremor
Secondary to drugs such as major tranquilizers, antipsychotics (including some of the new, atypical ones), and gastrointestinal motility agents	Symptoms begin on both sides of body; relatively rapid course with significant symptoms within one to two months; history of taking suspect medications
Dementia with Lewy bodies (diffuse Lewy body disease)	Parkinsonism plus prominent personality and cognitive problems; hallucinations can be troublesome
Alzheimer's disease	Personality changes and forgetfulness prominent and early, often associated with mild parkinsonism
Corticobasal degeneration (CBD)	Typically, markedly one-sided parkinsonism with jerky tremor-like movement (myoclonus) and difficulty using common objects

If you have been diagnosed with Parkinson's but observe that your symptoms are not characteristic of Parkinson's disease as described in this book, you may have another form of parkinsonism or a different type of disease altogether (Table 1.2) (see also Chapters 8, 9, and 10).

What Will Happen to Me If I Have Parkinson's?

Because Parkinson's disease is a progressive disorder, we can generally expect that each year the signs and symptoms of the disease will become more pronounced. With effective treatment, the symptoms may be so effectively masked that for some time it may seem that the disease is not changing, especially in the early years. Over time, however, even with treatment, most people who have Parkinson's do notice increasing problems. No one, not a physician or anyone else, can accurately predict how, or how quickly, the disease will progress in a specific individual. There simply is no reliable way to evaluate the degree of cell loss in the substantia nigra, no laboratory test or widely available imaging procedure that can tell us how much cell loss has occurred or how fast it is progressing. Even the new imaging techniques cannot predict severity or progression of disease.

We *can* say that Parkinson's is not the kind of disease in which, within a twelve-month period, someone who is able to walk and function independently suddenly finds herself or himself incapacitated and wheelchair-bound. In the average patient, the disorder is very slowly and gradually progressive over years, with relatively mild and subtle changes occurring in the first months to years of the illness.

Although we can't predict how the disease will progress in a specific individual, we do try to answer the questions patients naturally have about the course of their disease. Why? Because people need to know how long they can expect to remain employed or fully self-sufficient. They need to know how their disease will progress for financial, employment, and social planning reasons.

Disease progression varies greatly from one person to another. Some persons have a relatively rapid progression, beginning to experience significant physical disability within five years; others do not reach this state of disability for fifteen years. Sometimes these different disease courses are separated into "benign" and "malignant" forms. In our experience, most so-called malignant cases of Parkinson's disease have proved to be other diseases, which in their early stages were mimicking true Parkinson's disease (see Chapters 9 and 10).

A person's history with the disease is the best guide to the character of his or her illness in the future. In other words, a person's disease usually progresses at about the same rate that he or she has already experienced. This means that predictions are particularly difficult for people newly diagnosed with Parkinson's disease, because we have no information about how their disease has progressed so far. General information may be the best we can offer. In general, then, we say that when Parkinson's disease is diagnosed early, and when medications are used judiciously, people may experience five to ten years of motor symptoms that do not substantially interfere with their quality of life. Again, Parkinson's disease is not the kind of disease in which rapid deterioration occurs over a few months.

Although we do not yet have treatments capable of slowing or arresting the *progression* of the illness, current treatments can very effectively *relieve the symptoms,* especially in the early years. As mentioned, many persons who are adequately treated notice very little or no progression of symptoms over the first few years. Although we cannot slow the progression of the underlying illness, patients benefit greatly because reducing the symptoms delays disability in Parkinson's disease. However, with time, a person's degree of motor disability does tend to increase, and after five to ten years of illness the symptoms generally begin to disrupt daily life. At this point, medications are needed in higher doses and must be monitored and adjusted more frequently.

TREATMENT

Dramatic breakthroughs have been made in the management of Parkinson's disease, most notably the introduction of levodopa almost half a century ago and subsequently the use of dopamine agonists and, later, deep brain stimulation. As noted above, current treatment can significantly relieve people's symptoms, delay disability, and markedly improve their quality of life. Unfortunately, there is as yet no cure. (Treatment is discussed in more detail in Chapters 11 through 16.)

The first stage of treatment for Parkinson's is an accurate diagnosis. This is tricky, as we have noted, particularly early in the disorder when distinguishing Parkinson's disease from other diseases with similar symptoms is particularly difficult. It may be helpful to see a neurologist who is experienced with what are called *movement disorders*. A movement disorder specialist has expertise in diagnosing and treating Parkinson's disease and related disorders. A visit to a movement disorder center may also be useful. Most such centers are connected with a department of neurology at a medical school, although some are free-standing clinics. The centers have access to appropriate rehabilitation facilities and are usually involved in research studies.

We believe patients' involvement in research studies is a good idea, for several reasons. First, treatment of Parkinson's disease can be improved when people who have Parkinson's consent to participate in programs that test drugs, so there is an altruistic motive for some people. Second, in *clinical research trials,* new treatments are tested on patients in carefully planned studies designed or monitored by physicians and statisticians, and people in these trials might have access to helpful drugs years before the drugs are available to others. Finally, people who participate in clinical trials tend to do better than people who do not, even when the people in trials are receiving a placebo or "sugar pill" rather than a drug. This is because participants in clinical trials receive intense medical attention and monitoring; they are working with people who are especially interested in their disease; they are actively participating in controlling their disease; and they feel better. (See Chapter 18 for more information about medical research and clinical trials.)

You can find the names of movement disorder specialists by consulting Parkinson's disease patient organizations or by calling teaching hospitals associated with medical schools. Many of the Parkinson's disease Web sites for laypersons have lists of neurologists specializing in movement disorders. You can also write to the Movement Disorder Society or the American Academy of Neurology or go to their Web site (www .movementdisorders.org; www.aan.com) and get information on how to obtain the names of movement disorder specialists in your geographic region (see the Resources section at the end of the book).

Even if you live some distance from a specialist neurologist or specialist center, you may want to consider traveling to a specialist or center on one or more occasions for a confirming diagnosis, a second opinion, or a treatment plan. Often a specialist who is consulted in this way will remain available to your internist or your family doctor for consultation by telephone. For example, people living in, say, Montana, might, if they can afford it, go to the Mayo Clinic to visit a specialist. On returning home, care can generally be coordinated with a local neurologist or family doctor. Sometimes patients who live a long way from a specialist or center monitor their own symptoms and, rather than playing phone tag, they fax or email their questions to the specialist's office. The specialist then answers with recommendations. This is not the best possible system, but sometimes it is the best that can be managed. Increasingly, physicians and movement disorder centers are offering telemedicine care for patients living a long distance from the center. Find out whether this option is available in your area.

Patients who belong to a health maintenance organization (HMO) usually are obliged to use the HMO's doctors unless they get a special referral for someone outside the organization. The HMO may have its own neurologist. If you are in an HMO that does not have a neurologist, lobby firmly for a special referral.

WHEN SHOULD I TELL MY FAMILY, FRIENDS, AND COWORKERS?

As we note later in this book, family members—spouses, children, siblings—are often the first to notice symptoms in the person who has Parkinson's disease. They may notice a change in the way a person walks or stands or in the person's facial expression. But even if family members haven't yet noticed any symptoms in the person who has Parkinson's, they will notice them as time goes on. If you have been diagnosed with Parkinson's, rather than letting people close to you wonder and worry about what's wrong, it is generally best to tell them about the disease and that you are being treated for it. You can also assure them it is not a contagious disease and that except in a minority of families there is little evidence that it is passed from one generation to another.

Family members will share your concerns, of course, perhaps especially about the uncertainty of the future—the progression of the symptoms. But sharing your concerns as a family is almost always better than one person "braving it out" alone. And this way, too, the family can make plans for the future, perhaps taking that cross-country trip now rather than putting it off for years, as well as putting some savings away.

You would not be able to hide the symptoms of Parkinson's disease from your family indefinitely, and for this and these other reasons, our advice is to tell your family. Choose a place and time when you and they are comfortable, not stressed, and make sure you have lots of time to talk and share your feelings. If there are problems or tensions in your family that might make the telling difficult or even traumatic, you might want to enlist the help of a professional counselor or social worker, who can either advise you on how to break the news or be with you and your family during this time.

Deciding on the best time to tell an employer and colleagues about a Parkinson's diagnosis is often difficult. A person carrying a full load of responsibilities at work is naturally concerned that people will become uncertain about his or her ability to function if they learn about the diagnosis of a chronic illness. And people do sometimes react this way. Nonetheless, if you are in this situation, it is not a good idea to suppress information about your illness for too long. If your coworkers do not know about the disease, they might get some very wrong ideas: they might think the tremor means nervousness or anxiety, the masked face means boredom or displeasure, and the soft voice means a lack of conviction.

Parkinson's disease is a difficult disease to hide, anyway. People with a tremor would need to make up excuses about why their hand shakes. Or, if they tried to hide the tremor, they might become quite anxious, which makes the tremor worse. Most people decide it is just better to say, "I have Parkinson's."

Although Parkinson's is a fairly common disease, what most people "know" about it is often based on their experience with a relative or friend from some years ago. They probably aren't aware that the new medications are much better at managing the symptoms or that people who have the disease can continue to function well. So, once you make the decision to share this news with coworkers, keep in mind that they will react better to the news if you educate them a bit about how the disease does—and does not—affect you. When people who have Parkinson's were asked about their experience disclosing their diagnosis in the workplace, the majority reported that the news was received better than they expected.

There are other considerations. The federal Americans with Disabilities Act (ADA), signed into law in 1990, states that in a company with more than fifteen employees, the company is required to make "reasonable accommodations" in the workplace so that a person with a disability can continue to work. The ADA bans discrimination in employment against qualified persons with disabilities.

If oral presentations are a large part of your job, you may have difficulty if your voice becomes softer and more monotonous. Microphones and speaker systems can be used to make the presentations audible even to a large audience, however, so that your work can go on.

If you must have steady hands in your job, you may find your colleagues are alarmed by the tremor, even though it disappears when you are moving. You may need to explain about this aspect of tremor and demonstrate your abilities. Eventually, if tremor does become a problem, you may need to take on different tasks and responsibilities and give up tasks requiring a steady hand. Also, if stress and emotional intensity make the tremor worse, you may need to take care to avoid stressful situations.

The mood changes that sometimes appear early in Parkinson's may pose a problem for some people in a work situation. For example, someone with depression may find it very difficult to work effectively. Medical treatment of the depression generally helps with both the depression and effectiveness at work. A person who becomes unusually anxious in situations that previously would not have caused such distress may find medications can help relieve the anxiety (see Chapter 13). For many people, continuing to work and be productive is an important factor in adjusting to the diagnosis of Parkinson's disease. For others, symptoms such as fatigue and reduced tolerance to stress may make it difficult to cope with previous work demands, so approaches to work need to be individualized.

By now it is clear why patients and doctors alike understand that defining Parkinson's disease is both straightforward and elusive. The straightforward part is that we can describe Parkinson's disease as a specific neurologic disorder in which the destruction of specific centers within the brain disrupts people's control of movement. The disorder primarily involves a chemical deficiency of the neurotransmitter dopamine, and (as we'll discuss in Chapters 11 and 12) the replacement of dopamine significantly relieves the characteristic disease features of tremor, rigidity, slowness of movement, and difficulty with balance and posture.

What remains elusive is a precise definition and description of Parkinson's, as well as any understanding of its fundamental cause or causes. And progress of the disease varies significantly among people with the same signs and symptoms, and perhaps the same diagnosis, and we don't know why.

Here is the closest we can come to defining Parkinson's disease at this time: It is a slowly progressive neurodegenerative disease that has the characteristic "motor" symptoms of tremor, rigidity, slowness of movement, and gait and balance problems. Administering antiparkinson medications can relieve these symptoms. The degeneration in Parkinson's that accounts for many of the motor features occurs in the substantia nigra and the regions of the brain's motor control system downstream from the substantia nigra. A number of other diseases have some of these characteristics, but only Parkinson's disease has all of them. We also recognize that Parkinson's is more than a motor disorder and is more than a group of problems due to dopamine deficiency. As we learn more about the disease we hope to understand not only what causes it but how it can be treated more effectively and, someday, how it can be prevented.

In the next chapter we look at who gets Parkinson's disease; then we turn, in Chapter 3, to a description of the early symptoms.

CHAPTER 2

Who Gets Parkinson's Disease?

- *How common is Parkinson's disease?*
- *Is Parkinson's related to aging?*
- *Is it inherited?*
- *Is it triggered by environmental factors?*
- *What do we know about the causes of Parkinson's?*

When physicians make a diagnosis of any serious disease, patients and their families often ask, "Why me?" In the case of Parkinson's disease, the question "Why me?" is actually quite profound. The attempt to answer this question has occupied clinical researchers for many years.

The shortest and most direct answer is that, as of now, we don't know why one person develops Parkinson's and another does not. Science and medicine have told us some things about Parkinson's, but we still have much to learn. For example, although Parkinson's appears to be one of the most common neurodegenerative diseases in the United States and Canada, even after extensive studies we don't know for sure how many people have it, or who will get it, or why.

In this chapter we discuss what we do know and present some educated theories about why people get Parkinson's. First, though, it's helpful to consider the two major categories of all disease causation (what causes a particular disease)—genetic and environmental (nature and nurture). *Hereditary*, or *genetic*, diseases run in families and are passed from parent to child as part of the DNA, the genetic material that makes a person uniquely himself or herself. *Environmental* diseases are caused by something outside a person. This book considers environmental disease to be a disease caused by anything outside a person, anything other than a person's genetic material. Toxins, drugs, and even viruses or bacteria can be environmental causes of disease.

Even though the cause of Parkinson's remains elusive, in recent years there has been considerable interest in the possible role of genetics. The advances in technology allowing for more, and more sophisticated, examinations of the human genome result in more in-depth exploration of a possible genetic role in Parkinson's. During the same time, a number of population studies looking for environmental associations with the onset of Parkinson's have reported that exposure to herbicides and pesticides or certain solvents, frequency of bowel movements (although this could also be a very early feature of the disease), lower coffee consumption, smoking, and lower blood urate levels may somehow contribute to the development of the disease.

Most people who have Parkinson's cannot recall anyone else in their family having the disease, which would seem to rule out a very strong genetic cause in the majority of cases. And if environment were a cause, we might expect that persons married to each other for a long time and sharing a similar environment would both be affected by the disease—but such cases are rare.

The picture, then, is complex: Parkinson's disease may well be caused by a combination of genetic and environmental factors. Certain inherited characteristics might make it either more or less likely that a person will develop Parkinson's. For example, a person may inherit a predisposition to Parkinson's, but he or she will not develop the disease unless exposed to an environmental trigger of the disease, such as a toxin. Another person may have a genetic makeup that protects against Parkinson's even if she or he is exposed to the same toxin. Different combinations and amounts of genetic and environmental factors could also account for the differences between people's symptoms and the course of the disease.

Put another way, Person A, with genetic predisposition A and environmental trigger A, might have more severe Parkinson's symptoms than Person B, with genetic predisposition A and environmental trigger B. Person C might have a protective genetic component C and not get Parkinson's at all, even after exposure to triggers A or B. Other combinations of the above would yield different levels (or nonlevels) of disease.

Degenerative diseases usually are not caused by infections or metabolic disturbances or insufficient blood supply to the affected region (in this case, the substantia nigra). The cause of most neurodegenerative diseases remains unknown and is the focus of considerable research (see Chapter 18). Doctors and scientists are continuing to search for answers to the clearly complex question of what causes Parkinson's, and they will almost certainly succeed in unraveling some of the mysteries.

How Common Is Parkinson's?

Parkinson's disease is fairly common. A number of well-known people—many of whom are still working and changing the world—have been diagnosed with this disease. We estimate that, in North America, between 750,000 and a million people—slightly more men than women—have Parkinson's disease. For a variety of reasons, we don't know exactly how many. One reason is that many people are misdiagnosed: either their Parkinson's has not been recognized yet, or they have been diagnosed with Parkinson's but actually have some other disorder. And some people have not yet sought medical care for their symptoms. The best we can do is make estimates based on the widely varying results from door-to-door surveys, diagnoses of people admitted to hospitals, prescriptions for antiparkinson drugs, and information given on death certificates.

We also don't know whether Parkinson's is more common in some racial groups than in others. Several studies have suggested that the frequency of Parkinson's disease is higher in Caucasian American than in African American populations, but the results of these studies are difficult to accept. African Americans generally have less access than Caucasian Americans to medical care, particularly neurologic care, and accurate diagnosis of Parkinson's disease requires a person trained in and familiar with neurologic disorders. Thus, the reported racial differences may result from an inequality of medical care delivery in the United States. In one study at a specialized Parkinson's referral center in Baltimore, Maryland, African American Parkinson's patients were found to be visiting the center in small numbers, even though the city was home to a large population of African Americans. Further investigation showed that the African American patients generally visited the center at a more advanced stage of Parkinson's and that they had less access than other patients to the newer Parkinson's medications. Another study conducted a door-to-door survey in a multiracial county in Mississippi and found the frequency of Parkinson's disease in blacks and whites to be essentially the same. Other careful surveys indicate a higher occurrence of Parkinson's in Caucasians. In summary, the racial distribution of the disease remains unclear.

PARKINSON'S AND AGING

An actor wishing to portray an older person might move slowly and stoop over, assuming a flexed posture and perhaps shuffling along, and picking up things with trembling hands. The actor's use of features that commonly occur in Parkinson's disease both reflects the association between aging and Parkinson's in the actor's mind and reinforces this association in the popular imagination.

The average age of onset of Parkinson's disease is about sixty years. At the beginning of the twentieth century, sixty years seemed older than it does today and the average age of onset of Parkinson's was the same then as now. This may explain the long-held association between Parkinson's disease and aging. Now, though, we cannot say that Parkinson's affects only the elderly, although the number of people who have Parkinson's disease rises as the population ages: the chance of developing Parkinson's does increase as we age. Also, sixty is only the *average* age of onset. About 80 percent of all people who have Parkinson's develop the disorder between forty and seventy, and about 5 percent develop it between twenty and forty. The latter—so-called young-onset Parkinson's disease—is difficult to diagnose, primarily because neither physicians nor patients tend to think about Parkinson's disease in persons in their thirties (see Chapter 7).

The relationship between normal aging and the course and features of Parkinson's disease is hotly debated. Some researchers argue that everyone would eventually develop Parkinson's if they lived long enough because, in the normal process of aging, the dopamine-containing neurons of the substantia nigra, so essential for normal motor function, become dysfunctional and die. This position is not quite supported by the current evidence, which indicates that normal aging alone does not cause Parkinson's. It is true that once the substantia nigra is damaged by whatever does cause Parkinson's disease, the normal age-related loss of cells in the same area may contribute to the development of signs of the disease and possibly to its progression.

How much normal aging contributes to the signs, symptoms, and course of Parkinson's remains a hotly debated topic. However, age remains the most important risk factor for Parkinson's disease.

Is Parkinson's a Hereditary Disease?

As noted above, we do not know whether Parkinson's disease is inherited. For example, when a Parkinson's patient suggests the disease runs in his or her family and a neurologist trained in the diagnosis of movement disorders examines the affected family members, the neurologist often finds these family members have some other neurologic disorder, not Parkinson's disease. But we do know that if Parkinson's is diagnosed in one member of a family, there is a 10 to 15 percent chance that someone else in the family has Parkinson's as well. For most people who have Parkinson's, their family history has no pattern that suggests a genetic problem. When doctors inquire about genetic patterns of disease in a family, they are trying to determine whether certain well-known patterns of inheritance exist in that family—for example, are only members of one generation (siblings) affected (so-called recessive inheritance), or does the disease seem to pass from one generation to another (so-called dominant inheritance)? Even if in some families Parkinson's disease does occur in more than one generation or in brothers and sisters, we must remember that Parkinson's is common enough that coincidence might be playing a role.

Studies with identical twins seem to indicate that heredity alone does not cause Parkinson's in most patients. The medical profession considers such studies the best possible test—the gold standard—for determining whether a disease is genetic. Identical twins inherit the same genetic material, so if one twin develops a hereditary disease, the chances are very high that the other one will eventually develop it too. One very large National Institutes of Health study of Parkinson's disease identified forty-three identical twin pairs in which one twin had Parkinson's, as diagnosed by specially trained movement disorder experts. When these experts evaluated the other twin of each pair, they found that, among all forty-three pairs, only in one pair did both twins have Parkinson's. Two other twin studies, one in England and another in Finland, have reported similar findings.

This evidence indicates that inheritance probably does not play a predominant role in Parkinson's. The evidence was made stronger by the finding that even after reexamination of the twins some years later, when any previously unobserved Parkinson's symptoms should have surfaced, the incidence of both twins having Parkinson's disease remained extremely low.

A more recent twin study using a twin registry started by the federal government during World War II also demonstrated an extremely low occurrence of Parkinson's disease in both identical twins. Further, in this study the twins were examined at a much older age, so it is unlikely that a genetic influence on Parkinson's could have been missed. This study indicated that in patients with a younger age of onset, genetics did have a stronger role to play than in those with an older age of onset.

Even though it is still true that for an individual diagnosed with Parkinson's there is little chance of passing the disease to the next generation, we have learned a tremendous amount about genes and Parkinson's in the last ten years. When this new information began to emerge from laboratories around the world, the findings of abnormal genes in certain families with Parkinson's seemed unusual and difficult to understand. The developing story of the role of abnormal genes in Parkinson's has greatly increased our understanding of the basic chemical abnormalities in the brain in Parkinson's disease. The most important outcome of this new understanding is that it opens new avenues for pursuing better treatment for people who have Parkinson's. Some of these newly discovered "Parkinson's" genes are the α-synuclein gene, Parkin, DJ-1, PINK1, and LRRK2 as well as GBA, the gene known to cause Gaucher's disease.

The first Parkinson's disease gene was found in one very large Italian American family. In this family, almost half the children of any family member with Parkinson's will develop the disease. This extraordinary family can trace its history for many generations both in North America and in Italy, and these data allowed researchers to locate a genetic abnormality responsible for a type of Parkinson's disease.

The genetic abnormality in this family occurs in the α-synuclein gene, that is, the gene that directs the synthesis of α-synuclein, a brain protein located, among other places, in synaptic membranes—membranes vital to the transmission of chemical signals within the brain. Alpha-synuclein is also present in the abnormal cellular structures called Lewy bodies found in the brain cells of almost everyone with Parkinson's disease.

How relevant is this genetic abnormality to other people who have Parkinson's? Given that most patients' families reveal only weak or nonexistent familial patterns of Parkinson's disease and that this Italian family history is unusual, we don't know whether the abnormality is important to most people with the disease. In fact, scientists have failed to find this abnormal gene in most people who have typical Parkinson's disease. However, the importance of α-synuclein has been further confirmed by the findings that other mutations in the gene cause forms of parkinsonism and that the presence of too much of the gene (and thus the protein) also causes disease, with the amount of the excess gene (and protein) being related to the severity of the disease.

The second gene discovered, the Parkin gene, is responsible for a form of young-onset parkinsonism. It was first discovered in Japan, but researchers have since found this gene in various populations around the world. Although at first considered rare, it is now known to probably occur in approximately 10 percent of people whose disease began before age forty. It is becoming apparent that genetic influence in families is more likely if the person who has Parkinson's in that family has an early age of onset (usually before forty years old).

Other new genes discovered to play a role in families affected with Parkinson's include PINK1, DJ-1, LRRK2, GBA, and most recently VPS35. The LRRK2 gene has proved to be the most common known genetic cause of so-called dominantly inherited Parkinson's and has also been found in a small proportion of seemingly nonhereditary cases. ("Dominantly inherited" means that a characteristic is passed from parent to child 50 percent of the time, or, put another way, that a child has a one in two chance of inheriting it.) Additional genes associated with Parkinson's will certainly be discovered; using genome-wide association studies (GWAS, see below) a number of genes already have been found to possibly increase the risk of Parkinson's disease. All of these "new" Parkinson's genes are beginning to open up further areas of research that will ultimately lead to new treatments for symptoms and even to slowing the disease itself.

Scientists have learned about cell processes in Parkinson's disease that play an important role in how the disease evolves both in families with the abnormal gene and in patients with no family history of the disease. For example, the cellular process by which abnormal proteins in the cell are handled has become a focus of research. Some of the newly discovered genes help to regulate how these abnormally made cellular proteins are removed from the cell. One theory is that abnormal proteins inside the nerve cells of the substantia nigra and other brain areas cause these regions to degenerate and die. As we have discussed, when the substantia nigra degenerates, Parkinson's symptoms emerge. Researchers believe that the abnormal genes disrupt normal processes (carried out by cellular systems known as the ubiquitin-proteasome system and the lysosome-autophagy system) for removing "bad" or abnormal proteins. This removal process is very important to keeping nerve cells healthy.

It is now apparent that typical Parkinson's signs and symptoms—resting tremor, rigidity, slowness, gait and balance problems, good response to levodopa, the emergence of motor fluctuations and dyskinesias (discussed later), and unilateral onset—can be seen in genetically determined Parkinson's. This is an extraordinary discovery, and even though the overall percentage of families with these genetic abnormalities remains low, the fact that there are several different distinct genes that cause Parkinson's has awakened the research community to the vast possibilities that lie ahead to better understand the basic mechanisms responsible for Parkinson's disease and to create better treatments.

These new genetic discoveries combined with the rapidly advancing technology used in genetic analysis has led to the beginning of a technique known as GWAS (genome-wide association studies). In these studies, the entire human genome is looked at for clues to the cause of Parkinson's. Even more exciting is the use of gene-sequencing techniques, which are becoming more widely available and will allow an individual patient's genome to be analyzed to look for clues into the origin of their Parkinson's.

In addition to the traditional forms of inheritance, which we have already discussed—dominant (generation to generation) and recessive (siblings only)—these new techniques and studies allow the research field to expand into examining Parkinson's as a "complex" genetic disorder in which it may be found that one abnormal gene is not responsible for the clinical symptoms of Parkinson's; rather, arrays of genes may be involved, with each individual gene exerting only a very small effect. When the necessary array of ten, twenty, forty genes is aligned, this may trigger Parkinson's.

Although the evidence in recent years has grown stronger that Parkinson's is a complex genetic disorder, environmental triggers have not been eliminated as a potential factor. As an example of this, consider that if a person carries the LRRK2 gene, it does not mean that the person will develop Parkinson's. There are examples of people living to a very elderly age with the LRRK2 gene who never develop Parkinson's. The reason for this is not certain. Is it because the secondary array of "genes" was not sufficient to trigger Parkinson's, or because the individual never came into contact with some unknown environmental triggering factor?

As scientists continue to explore these new avenues of research, we will learn more and more about the fundamental chemical problems both in Parkinson's in families with abnormal genes and in more typical, nonfamilial Parkinson's. This will be the beginning of a vast new understanding of the molecular basis of Parkinson's disease.

ENVIRONMENTAL FACTORS AND PARKINSON'S

When patients diagnosed with Parkinson's ask "Why me?" they are often wondering whether they have been exposed to "something" that could have triggered their disease. Here is what we know about the influence of environmental toxins, drugs, or viruses or bacteria on the development of Parkinson's disease.

Industrial Toxins

The evidence shows a "definite maybe" for the possibility of environmental toxins as a cause of Parkinson's disease. A number of toxins, including manganese dust, carbon disulfide, and carbon monoxide, have been shown to cause parkinsonism, but not, according to research so far, Parkinson's disease.

Although the symptoms of Parkinson's disease have distinctive, easily recognized characteristics, there is a surprising absence of mention of these symptoms in the medical literature before James Parkinson's 1817 paper. In part because of this, the theory has been advanced that the frequency of Parkinson's has increased since the industrial revolution. If this intriguing idea were to prove true, perhaps Parkinson's could be related to some type of industrial toxin. However, we know that the frequency of Parkinson's disease has not changed from the late 1890s to the present—a period of rapid increase in industrialization—and this would seem to argue against industrial toxins as an important causative factor. In addition, there are very clear older descriptions of Parkinson's disease, including writings from ancient Egypt.

The idea that industrialization might increase the incidence of Parkinson's disease also suggests that city dwellers, who are more likely than country dwellers to be exposed to certain industrial pollutants, might also be more likely to develop Parkinson's. Some reports show that city dwellers may well have a higher frequency, but even more studies suggest that rural life predisposes individuals to Parkinson's disease. Country life may entail different environmental exposures, such as to substances found in some well water. Again, the evidence is unclear.

Environmental studies are difficult to design and carry out with accuracy. Many environmental studies are still under way and may yet reveal the cause of Parkinson's disease, but, as interesting as these conclusions would be, this research is still a work in progress. Sometimes the media report that a specific toxin might be the cause of Parkinson's, and people become concerned. In every case thus far, repeated studies of the same toxin have not supported the earlier findings. A current source of such controversy is the potential for welding to cause Parkinson's disease.

Illicit Drugs

A number of years ago, a tragic error in the home production of a mind-altering drug provided some intriguing evidence about how environmental toxins might cause parkinsonism. Young drug users were making a drug called meperidine, which was supposed to produce a euphoric altered state of consciousness. They made a mistake in their preparation, however, and produced a heroin-like compound called MPTP (methyl phenyl tetrahydropyridine). This substance is capable of causing sudden and dramatic injury to the dopamine-producing cells of the substantia nigra. Some of the young people who injected the drug intravenously suddenly (within two to four weeks) developed the symptoms of advanced Parkinson's.

This tragedy has spawned numerous scientific studies, as scientists seek to understand *how* MPTP injures nerve cells and whether other, similar substances are present in our environment. After decades of exploration of MPTP-induced injury of dopamine cells in animal models, this paradigm is being critically reevaluated. Although these studies have been very helpful in understanding the brain's response to dopaminergic injury, the translation of the results of these experiments into clinical trials has been disappointing. In other words, studies of animals subjected to MPTP injury and then treated with another drug to dampen the injury (sometimes called "neuroprotection") have been successfully conducted. Unfortunately, when these drugs were tried in patients with early Parkinson's to slow progression, all of them failed. This has led to a search for better animal models of Parkinson's. (See Chapter 9 for further information on MPTP.)

The Roles of Viruses or Bacteria

There is no evidence that Parkinson's disease results directly from infection with any type of virus or bacteria. Sometimes, but very rarely, a person who has had encephalitis (a brain infection caused by a large variety of viruses) develops parkinsonism, but the symptoms usually fade within a few days or a month.

Historically, though, we can find some evidence for a possible virus-associated parkinsonism. During the influenza pandemic of 1917 to 1920, a particular type of parkinsonism developed in people who had a disease called von Economo's encephalitis. Some of these people suddenly (overnight) developed what we now call parkinsonism, and some developed it two or three years later. Unlike people who have more typical postencephalitic parkinsonism, these patients did not get better. In general, although encephalitis can cause parkinsonism, it does not cause true Parkinson's. Postencephalitic parkinsonism was well portrayed in Oliver Sacks's book *Awakenings*, which was subsequently made into an award-winning movie.

No evidence suggests that Parkinson's disease is contagious. A person who cares for or lives with someone with Parkinson's has no more risk of developing the disease than the general population.

How Could Factors outside the Body Trigger Parkinson's Symptoms?

Even if we do not know what causes Parkinson's, it would be useful to know the mechanism by which anything could cause it. How could an environmental factor cause Parkinson's disease? There are many theories. For example, if a developing fetus is exposed to a toxin, the infant might have fewer than the normal number of neurons in the substantia nigra. This might leave a sufficient number of neurons for normal motor development and normal motor behavior during the first few decades of life, but the shortage of neurons could eventually cause symptoms as dopamine-producing cells were lost during the normal aging process. A similar mechanism might underlie a loss of substantia nigra neurons later in life that, while not causing symptoms at the time of the loss, might cause them as aging progresses.

In another scenario, a series of exposures to a toxin over time might repeatedly injure the neurons, producing a later decline in the total number of substantia nigra neurons. Although each single exposure

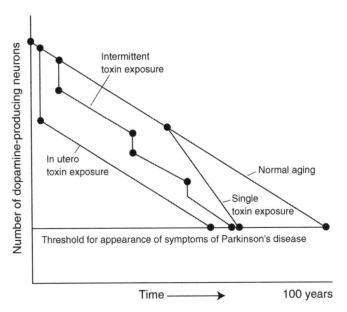

FIGURE 2.1 This diagram illustrates potential ways in which exposure to various environmental or endogenous toxins might result in the appearance of Parkinson's disease. The symptoms and signs of Parkinson's disease begin to emerge in people when 70 to 80 percent of dopaminergic neurons in the substantia nigra are nonfunctional. Some authorities believe that if everyone lived long enough, normal aging and subsequent loss of dopamine neurons would result in the symptoms of Parkinson's disease in all people. In the figure this concept is labeled *normal aging*. The diagram is theoretical and suggests that by age one hundred symptoms of Parkinson's disease might develop in all of us. The *other lines* on the diagram indicate ways in which single intermittent or even in utero toxin exposure might harm dopamine neurons and eventually result in the appearance of symptoms of Parkinson's disease.

might not be enough to cause symptoms, the accumulated losses, along with the normal aging process, could ultimately lead to the onset of disease.

Also plausible is a mechanism in which a toxin might activate a steady and unnaturally rapid decline in cell numbers over many years. The loss of enough cells could push the brain over the threshold of "normal" and produce the symptoms we know as Parkinson's disease (Figure 2.1). However, all of these hypotheses need to take into account that Parkinson's involves far more than the dopamine cells in the substantia nigra.

At present, the most widely touted hypothesis explaining the development of Parkinson's disease combines exposure to environmental factors with genetic predisposing factors. Perhaps certain environmental factors affect only those people who have some sort of inherited susceptibility to them. We may find that multiple environmental factors injure these cells and that no single, specific, toxin is responsible for Parkinson's disease.

Along the same lines, there may be multiple genetic predisposing factors. Every person may represent a variable combination of environmental and genetic factors. The heavier the load of these factors, the greater is the likelihood of developing the disease. It is also possible that protective genetic factors could reduce the risk of specific environmental factors (i.e., the opposite of genetic predisposition).

We have only these pieces of evidence and hypotheses with which to respond to the newly diagnosed person's compelling question of "Why me?" So far we have no satisfactory answer. When we are able to answer this question, we will be close to understanding the cause of Parkinson's disease. One important consideration is that there is likely no single cause; it may be more appropriate for us to think in terms of Parkinson's diseases rather than considering it a single uniform disease entity.

Part II

Signs and Symptoms of Parkinson's Disease

CHAPTER 3

Early Symptoms

- *What symptoms might appear even before a doctor can diagnose Parkinson's disease?*
- *What symptoms are common, yet often go unrecognized, as features of the disease?*

It is often difficult to pinpoint when a person who has Parkinson's first began showing signs and symptoms of the disease. Many people vividly recall when they first noticed their tremor, but through close questioning, the physician often finds that subtle signs of the disease were present even before the tremor became noticeable.

When these early symptoms first appear, they may be similar to symptoms of other disorders and thus not useful as signposts either toward or away from Parkinson's, and they often are not very helpful in early diagnosis. People who consult a physician about very early, mild symptoms of Parkinson's may be frustrated with the medical profession for a while, because doctors often cannot make a quick diagnosis. Some patients have the sense that the cause of their symptoms is being overlooked, and they visit a variety of health-related professionals in search of a definitive diagnosis. This is understandable, but the fact is that diagnosing Parkinson's based on very early symptoms is seldom possible.

After a physician suspects Parkinson's, however, looking back at these early symptoms can help confirm or dismiss the diagnosis. Once the diagnosis of Parkinson's is made, many patients express relief that this period of uncertainty has been resolved.

TABLE 3.1
EARLY SIGNS AND SYMPTOMS OF PARKINSON'S DISEASE

Change in facial expression (staring, lack of blinking)
Failure to swing one arm when walking
Flexion (stooped) posture
"Frozen," painful shoulder
Limping or dragging of one leg
Numbness, tingling, achiness, or discomfort of the neck or limbs
Loss of sense of smell
Softness of the voice
Subjective sensation of internal trembling
Resting tremor

Table 3.1 summarizes some signs and symptoms of early Parkinson's disease.

SYMPTOMS ON ONE SIDE ONLY

For unknown reasons, the symptoms of early Parkinson's commonly begin on one side of the body. For example, one leg may be affected while the other leg remains unaffected for two or more years. People sometimes wonder whether the side of onset of the symptoms has any relationship to handedness, but no such connection has been established. Physicians who have little experience with Parkinson's may not be aware that the occurrence of early symptoms on only one side of the body is very typical of the disease.

INTERNAL TREMOR

Early on, many persons who have Parkinson's notice an internal tremor, a feeling of trembling within a limb or their trunk. Nearly half of our patients report feeling that one of their legs or arms, or their abdomen, is trembling, yet neither the patient nor the doctor can see any movement. An internal tremor is likely to be a Parkinson's-induced tremor that has acquired adequate force for the person to feel it but not enough force to cause visible movement. The presence of an internal tremor can help the doctor make a diagnosis, so it's important to report any sensation of internal tremor.

MILD TREMOR

When someone experiences an involuntary, mild tremor that is characteristic of early Parkinson's, some physicians may dismiss it as a sign of anxiety or aging. Patients also may report a mild, intermittent tremor along with a variety of vague symptoms including fatigue, weakness, muscle aches, impaired concentration, and sleep disturbance. These symptoms are also characteristic of depression and anxiety (as discussed later in this chapter), however, so physicians sometimes have difficulty knowing what is causing them.

EMOTIONAL EFFECTS

The Parkinson's tremor becomes more intense with any kind of strong emotion, including sexual arousal. Sometimes people become alarmed by this and think it means their Parkinson's is getting worse. This is not so. As soon as their emotional level, or arousal, returns to normal, so does the tremor. These patients can be reassured that sexual relations generally are part of a warm, supportive relationship and should be continued.

PAIN AND OTHER SENSORY EFFECTS

Early Parkinson's disease may cause a variety of aches and pains around the neck, shoulders, arms, legs, or lower back. Many people have such pains, so part of the doctor's task is to distinguish between ordinary occasional pain and pain caused by Parkinson's. On the side first affected by Parkinson's, about 10 percent of patients develop a painful, stiff shoulder called *frozen shoulder*. Sometimes this is the first sign that something is wrong with arm function. Frozen shoulder is caused by the slowly increasing symptoms of rigidity and slowness; these symptoms, in turn, gradually restrict the range of normal movement of the shoulder joint. One way a doctor can tell whether shoulder, neck, or arm pain is caused by Parkinson's is by finding whether the pain is alleviated by antiparkinson medication. Aches and pains resulting from muscle stiffness and rigidity can be alleviated when appropriate antiparkinson medication is taken (see Chapter 4). On the other hand, a frozen shoulder resulting from early Parkinson's may in addition require physical therapy to mobilize the shoulder and relieve pain.

People also report other sensory effects associated with Parkinson's disease. They frequently describe sensations of numbness, tingling, burning, coldness, or aching in their arms, legs, back, abdomen, or pelvic regions. These sensations generally come and go—they are not constant. Sometimes they occur when the antiparkinson medication is working, but more often when it is not. Although these sensory phenomena are usually not disabling, they can be disruptive and uncomfortable.

The sense of smell, or olfaction, is one of our "special senses." A reduced or lost sense of smell is a common feature in Parkinson's disease, even very early in the course. Loss of the sense of smell is most commonly recognized as a changed perception in how food tastes. Smell is very closely associated with taste, and people may report that their favorite foods do not "taste" right. Many people who have Parkinson's, in retrospect, recall noting loss of their sense of smell well before other symptoms developed. However, this is a nonspecific symptom that can be caused by many other factors—repeated nasal infections, smoking, head injury, and other causes.

FOOT CRAMPS

Occasionally, in early Parkinson's, people notice early morning foot cramps, which may or may not be painful. These cramps are known as *dystonic spasm* or *dystonia* (*dys* meaning "bad" or "incorrect," and *tonic* referring to muscle tone). All the toes may curl downward, or the big toe may bend up while the other toes curl down. Much less often, the hand may be affected in a similar way, usually when the person is engaged in activities such as writing, so the fingers or wrist assume an abnormal posture (see below and Chapter 4).

MASKED FACIAL EXPRESSION

Early in the disease, family members may notice changes in the person's facial expression. Doctors use the term *masked face* to describe the loss of spontaneous facial expression and the decreased frequency of blinking that make people who have Parkinson's appear to be staring. Physicians may misinterpret this lack of facial animation as evidence of depression, and family members or friends may think that the patient is disinterested, unengaged, or unhappy, but in fact it is caused by the Parkinson's rigidity and slowing of the muscles, particularly those that produce facial expression and blinking.

VOICE CHANGES

People who have Parkinson's often report that their voice has lost its "power" and that they have to work hard to maintain the volume of their speech. Husbands or wives often observe that their spouse's voice has become softer, perhaps so soft that they must frequently ask him or her to repeat things. (Sometimes this triggers a charge by the spouse with Parkinson's that the husband's or wife's hearing is declining and, if in fact this is the case, communication can become even more challenging.) People who have Parkinson's disease may be particularly difficult to understand on the telephone. In the workplace, they may have difficulty expressing their ideas at meetings or when giving formal presentations.

LOSS OF HAND DEXTERITY

Because Parkinson's affects the fluidity and rapidity of movements, routine tasks involving hand dexterity often feel awkward as symptoms begin to emerge. People may begin to have a difficult time using the computer keyboard, or they may feel clumsy when taking their keys or wallet out of a pocket.

Many people with early symptoms have difficulty with the flow of

FIGURE 3.1 Handwriting of a person who has Parkinson's, illustrating micrographia.

their handwriting, particularly if the symptoms begin on their dominant side (right side for a right-hander). People report that their handwriting is slower and more laborious, and that the words start out normal-sized then gradually shrink; this tiny handwriting is called *micrographia* (Figure 3.1). If you look at people's signatures over the years—for example, on their credit card receipts or checks—you may be able to see a pattern of progressive micrographia.

People need fine dexterity to fasten a top shirt button or apply makeup, and difficulties with these tasks may show up early in the disease. If, as often occurs, one side is affected before the other, the person may have trouble buttoning one shirtsleeve but not the other. Tasks that require repetitive, rotary motions at the wrist, such as beating eggs or brushing teeth, can also be difficult as early symptoms appear. Patients often interpret these problems as being due to "weakness," and when tremor is absent their physician might consider such "weakness" on one side of the body as a possible symptom of a stroke or a tumor affecting the opposite side of the brain.

Stooped Posture

Mild stooping of posture can be observed in the early stages of Parkinson's disease. People who have Parkinson's may become increasingly stooped or bent over with time. Such stooping can be a normal sign of aging, so by itself it does not provide enough evidence for a doctor to diagnose Parkinson's disease.

Difficulties in Walking and Other Whole Body Movements

Changes in arm movements when walking are subtle, but people who have Parkinson's and their family members often notice these changes early on. Normally, we spontaneously swing our arms in an alternating manner when we walk. In early Parkinson's, natural arm swing is often lost on one side. Some people say their arm seems to be stuck at their side when they walk, or that it seems to stay slightly bent or flexed at the elbow and doesn't swing naturally when they walk. When they think about it, they can swing the arm, but it returns to its immobile state at their side if they stop making this conscious effort.

Similarly, when one leg no longer moves fluidly, some people feel as if that leg is dragging behind. The rhythm of their gait may alter, and they may show a slight limp.

Mostly because of the slowness of movement in Parkinson's, people who have early disease also may find it increasingly difficult to get out of low, soft chairs or sofas. Getting in and out of an automobile can also be more difficult.

Loss of Balance

Postural reflex is the term used to describe the many reflexes necessary to maintain balance when standing or walking. Although loss of balance and falling are rarely a problem until late in the course of Parkinson's, some people develop unsteadiness early in the course of the disease. When a person loses balance and falls before the onset of any symptoms and signs typical of true Parkinson's disease, this often indicates some other disease, possibly one of the diseases that mimics Parkinson's (see Chapter 10).

People who have Parkinson's may have a subtle feeling of not being steady on their feet, and they may have difficulty turning around rapidly. Their imbalance may cause difficulty in standing on one foot to pull on trousers or put on socks or stockings. The imbalance may be more noticeable when they are walking on an uneven surface or rising from a couch or an awkward position (e.g., while gardening). In advanced stages of Parkinson's, balance problems may become serious enough that a person will fall without any obvious reason, such as light-headedness or double vision (see Chapters 4 and 5).

As noted above, a history of early falling is usually not associated with typical Parkinson's disease. Physicians take this problem very seriously, though, and instruct their medical students and neurology residents that adults do not repeatedly fall down without a reason.

DEPRESSION

Receiving a diagnosis of Parkinson's disease is difficult, and the news often leads to a normal stage of transient depression and grief over the loss of health. People may be so focused on their concern about their health and their future that they lose interest in other things for a while. Sometimes they have difficulty seeing ahead to a time when these feelings will subside, but with time, as people gradually accept their disorder, many of these feelings *will* pass.

Severe, persistent depression is quite different from these feelings related to the news about one's health. It is a serious illness requiring medical attention. A person affected by this type of depression has pervasive feelings of sadness and hopelessness, along with a number of other symptoms, including feeling overwhelmed, feeling afraid, being anxious, not being able to make decisions, having little energy, and taking little pleasure in things that used to be of interest (apathy); sleep disturbances (too much or too little sleep); appetite disturbances (increased or decreased); and vague aches and pains.

Depression brought on by a life event, such as a diagnosis of Parkinson's disease, is sometimes called *reactive depression* or *secondary depression*. This is different from endogenous depression, or *primary depression*, which seems to arise suddenly, with no clear cause.

While depression can be an early symptom of Parkinson's, few physicians recognize it as such. Depression is common throughout the population, affecting men and women of all ages and racial groups. Furthermore, some symptoms of depression overlap with those of Parkinson's disease. Slowness of movement and loss of facial animation, for example, are symptoms of both depression and Parkinson's. A variety of vague symptoms, including fatigue, weakness, muscle aches, impaired concentration, and sleep disturbance, may occur in people who have depression or Parkinson's. Depression can be misdiagnosed as Parkinson's, and vice versa. In other words, a thorough history and examination are needed to sort out what is causing these symptoms. After Parkinson's has progressed, one can often look back and see that depression was one of the initial symptoms.

Doctors often see people who have Parkinson's who have noticed significant changes of mood and behavior for some time before they suspected Parkinson's disease or before a diagnosis of Parkinson's was made. Again, it is important to distinguish between the symptoms of Parkinson's disease and the symptoms of depression. For example, a depressed person, like a person who has early Parkinson's, may show a loss of facial expression, slowed movement, and a stooping posture, and may speak in a low monotone. People who have Parkinson's disease may also notice they have less interest in hobbies that used to be a source of particular enjoyment—as do people who have depression. An anxious patient may feel tremulous, a feeling similar to the internal tremor or early tremor of Parkinson's.

People who have Parkinson's who are still in the workplace may find themselves having unaccustomed difficulties with their oral presentations or sales techniques. Such difficulties may be due to Parkinson's-related voice changes, but patients or their doctors may attribute the difficulties to emerging anxiety accompanied by social phobia. Retired individuals may describe an unusual hesitation or discomfort in social situations and attribute it to retirement rather than to Parkinson's disease or depression.

People whose Parkinson's symptoms include depression generally find their depression continues. There are many treatments for depression, though, and many of these therapies are effective for people who have Parkinson's (see Chapter 13).

ANXIETY

As we've already noted, people who have Parkinson's may find they are more anxious, nervous, and agitated in situations that would not have bothered them before. Some anxiety may be a reaction to symptoms of Parkinson's, such as tremor or difficulty with speech. People who have Parkinson's may also be concerned about what others will think if they shake, have trouble speaking in public, or are unable to walk normally. Some emotional distress appears to be a result of the deterioration of the dopamine system.

General anxiety, social phobia, and panic attacks all can be associated with Parkinson's disease. A person who has *social phobia* experiences anxiety and discomfort in settings requiring interactions with others. For example, this may occur in the workplace when an individual experiences uncharacteristic difficulty making a sales pitch, participating in a meeting, or giving a public address. People may also suddenly find they are uncomfortable at social gatherings or entertaining friends and family in their home.

Panic attacks are acute episodes of severe anxiety. They may be triggered by stressful events or they may come out of nowhere. They're extremely frightening: the individual is suddenly hit with severe anxiety and a sense of impending doom. During a panic attack, a person may experience a rapid heartbeat, tremulousness, and perspiration.

Fortunately, both social phobia and panic attacks usually respond well to medication, especially the selective serotonin reuptake inhibitors (SSRIs), discussed further in Chapter 13.

Apathy

Some people who have Parkinson's lose their motivation to pursue old activities or start new ones, and they may become socially withdrawn. This apathy may be associated with depression or may even be a sign of developing dementia. Unfortunately, current drugs are not as effective as we would like in treating apathy (see Chapter 6).

Fatigue

Fatigue is another common symptom of Parkinson's disease that may occur in the early stages of the illness. Fatigue needs to be distinguished from apathy, depression, and excessive sleepiness, all of which may be due to the disease or in some cases to a complication of certain treatments (especially sleepiness). Fatigue may improve with medication for Parkinson's but it often persists and represents a challenge to our current treatments (see Chapter 6).

Is There a "Parkinsonian Personality"?

A fair amount of discussion has occurred on whether or not there is a parkinsonian personality. This question is very interesting, if exceedingly hypothetical. The real interest here relates to the question of whether the incubation time for Parkinson's disease is long or short.

According to the standard description, people who have Parkinson's tend to be very strict, rule-abiding citizens, who do not smoke or drink and are particularly straitlaced in social mores. This is obviously an over-simplification of a very complex issue. Many people who have Parkinson's disease do not display these traits at all. But might some combination of personality traits tie in with an incubation period for Parkinson's disease before any symptoms appear?

If there is a parkinsonian tendency toward certain traits, perhaps the disease process affects behavior for years and decades before any noticeable sign of the disease. More recent scientific investigations using special imaging systems such as positron emission tomography (PET) and single photon emission computed tomography (SPECT) suggest the existence of a presymptomatic period of approximately five years and perhaps longer during which the disease process has started but the person feels or experiences no obvious symptoms that can be clearly attributed to the disease. When researchers eventually develop drugs to prevent or slow the progression of Parkinson's disease, great emphasis will be placed on ways of identifying persons who have preclinical (presymptomatic) disease.

Early Diagnosis Is Difficult

No definitive laboratory test or radiologic study is available for diagnosing Parkinson's disease, so the diagnosis must be based on the clinical judgment of the physician, piecing together historical clues and findings from a thorough physical examination. This remains true even with the advent of the dopamine transporter scan (SPECT) (see Chapter 8). Parkinson's is a serious disease, and its treatment involves some serious choices about medications, so no physician is comfortable rushing into a diagnosis of Parkinson's. Because the initial symptoms can be very subtle and may be overlooked or mistaken for other medical problems, a firm diagnosis is difficult in the early stages. Sometimes the only way to differentiate Parkinson's from these other diseases is to wait and see whether the typical Parkinson's symptoms get worse.

In our practice, when we are undecided about a serious neurologic disorder such as Parkinson's disease, we often ask the patient to return after three to six months so we can see whether the subtle signs have progressed, new signs have developed, and the signs or symptoms characteristic of Parkinson's have appeared. People are understandably frustrated with this delay, but often it is the only way to diagnose accurately. In these instances, the question will arise about the utility of a SPECT Scan, but these scans cannot diagnose Parkinson's. The SPECT Scan can tell us whether or not there is a detectable alteration in the dopamine system, but even if an alteration is seen, a diagnosis of Parkinson's is not certain (see Chapter 8).

A physician who diagnoses Parkinson's disease should have expertise in neurologic diagnosis. If you have Parkinson's-like symptoms, you should consult a neurologist, or even a neurologist who is an expert in the diagnosis and management of movement disorders. As noted in Chapter 1, movement disorder specialists and neurologists at centers for the study of movement disorders have special training in diagnosing and treating people who experience problems with odd movements. (See Chapter 1 for suggestions on how to locate specialists and specialist centers.)

As the symptoms of Parkinson's disease increase in severity, a definitive diagnosis can usually be made and medications can be prescribed to help the person continue functioning. This stage of Parkinson's disease, called moderate Parkinson's disease, is discussed in the next chapter.

CHAPTER 4

Moderate Parkinson's Disease

- *What are the characteristic symptoms of moderate Parkinson's disease?*
- *Which symptoms respond well to medication, and which symptoms are more difficult to treat?*
- *What other, less common, symptoms might occur in moderate Parkinson's?*

In this chapter we describe the motor symptoms of moderate Parkinson's disease (the TRAP symptoms, as described in Chapter 1) and the most common nonmotor symptoms associated with this stage of Parkinson's. We begin with the motor symptoms.

MOTOR SYMPTOMS OF MODERATE PARKINSON'S DISEASE

Tremor

Tremor, or involuntary rhythmic shaking, of the hand, foot, or regions around the mouth is without doubt the most common symptom and sign of Parkinson's disease, although some patients with Parkinson's never develop a tremor. Seventy-five percent of all patients with Parkinson's begin their illness with the emergence of tremor. It is most likely to start in a hand or arm, although a leg may also be affected and, far less frequently, the face.

The Parkinson's tremor, commonly referred to as *resting tremor*, has very specific characteristics and tends to be most severe when a person's hands are completely at rest. The tremor usually diminishes and may entirely disappear when the hands are moving as the person engages in tasks such as reaching for a cup, holding a fork, or writing. Even people who have a moderate to severe resting tremor often find their tremor is markedly reduced when they fasten buttons or place pen to paper, although holding the limb in a particular position is often associated with the tremor coming out again or reemerging.

As noted in Chapter 3, very early in the disease, tremor may be internal, with no movement visible to doctor or patient. People who have Parkinson's may first notice the resting tremor when they are sitting with their hands in their lap or when they are walking with their arms hanging naturally at their sides. Others may notice that their thumb and fingers tremble when they sit quietly reading the newspaper or lost in thought while gazing at a computer screen. Sometimes the visible tremor starts with involuntary movements of the fingers and thumb, perhaps similar to rolling a marble between thumb and forefinger. A tremor may also involve repetitive rotating movements of the wrist or movements of the toes or ankles, and occasionally movement around the lips.

As we also noted in Chapter 3, a tremor almost always begins on one side of the body. With time, this unilateral tremor frequently evolves into a tremor affecting both sides. The tremor tends to start out focused on one part of the body, such as in a finger, then invariably progresses to other areas on the same side of the body. For example, if a tremor starts with the right hand, it is more likely to spread to the right leg before affecting any part of the left side of the body. Initially, a tremor may be intermittent or even fleeting and appear only in response to stress or fatigue. With time, however, it becomes more noticeable and more pronounced during a person's waking hours.

At any stage of Parkinson's disease, the tremor varies over the course of the day. Emotional states and variations in sleep patterns have a profound influence on tremors. Emotional excitement, whether stemming from anger, anxiety, enthusiasm, or sexual arousal, often makes the tremor worse.

While this experience may be frightening, the worsening of a tremor is only temporary and in no way alters the course of Parkinson's disease. People who have Parkinson's sometimes believe that because excitement makes their tremor worse, they must try to avoid becoming upset or excited as part of controlling their illness. This is not true—fortunately, since it would be an impossible task. When people who have Parkinson's return to their more ordinary emotional state, their tremor likewise returns to its "normal" level. Although elevated emotional states do cause a mild tremor to become moderate or a moderate tremor to become severe, increased intensity of tremor lasts only roughly as long as the state of emotional excitement.

Tremor is also affected by sleep. When people who have Parkinson's are fully asleep, their tremor entirely subsides. Within moments of waking up (or shortly before), however, the tremor reappears. Sleep is thus associated with the waxing and waning of a tremor. Some consider this variation in tremor as evidence that the tremor is of psychiatric origin. This notion, of course, is patently false. All patients and physicians familiar with Parkinson's disease recognize the profound influence of sleep, arousal, and emotional states on the expression of Parkinson's-related tremor.

For some people who have Parkinson's disease, the tremor is a disturbing symptom that may cause them to feel extremely embarrassed or ashamed to be seen in public. If you have a tremor that makes you uncomfortable in social situations or causes you psychological distress, this may be a reason to initiate or change medical treatments.

Although a tremor can become something of a disability as it interferes with daily activities, it is usually not incapacitating. Tremor is usually more of a nuisance, and one that tends to draw unwanted attention from observers. Some people who have Parkinson's focus on the tremor as their central problem, but the real cause of difficulties with hand dexterity is increased rigidity and slowness of movement. Outcome studies (clinical research that follows the effects of certain Parkinson's symptoms on disability) have shown that of all the symptoms and signs of Parkinson's, tremor is the least likely to result in disability. It can also sometimes be more resistant to medical therapy than other early features.

Rigidity

People with Parkinson's rarely go to their doctor's office complaining of rigidity, even though it causes stiffness of muscles and may be responsible for increasing neck, back, and limb pain, hand awkwardness, and clumsiness. During a physical examination, a doctor tests muscle tone by flexing and extending the patient's arms and legs to check for excessive rigidity.

Two types of rigidity are associated with Parkinson's disease. Parkinson's can produce *lead pipe rigidity,* a smooth resistance that feels to the examining doctor like the resistance to bending a soft lead pipe. Alternatively, a person who has Parkinson's may have *cogwheel rigidity,* which the doctor feels as a ratchet-like increase in tone reminiscent of a turning cogwheel as he or she bends the patient's elbow back and forth or moves a wrist up and down. Cogwheel rigidity suggests the presence of an underlying tremor, even if it is not visible. A physician can feel it at the neck, in the upper extremities, and occasionally in the lower extremities.

Foot Cramps

Foot and leg cramps in Parkinson's disease, called *dystonic spasm,* may or may not be painful. The cramps are muscle spasms that often pull the foot into abnormal postures. The toes may curl down while the big toe curls upward, or the foot may turn in at the ankle—or all of these things may happen together. The spasms make walking difficult and are often uncomfortable or even extremely painful.

The cramps seem to occur most frequently when medication levels are low, such as upon arising in the morning. Often the foot cramp subsides following the morning dose of antiparkinson medication, but it may return intermittently during the day. The cramps may be eased by switching to a long-acting preparation of antiparkinson drugs or by taking another dose part way through the night.

Akinesia or Bradykinesia

The slowness of movement in Parkinson's disease, called *bradykinesia,* begins almost imperceptibly, producing subtle awkwardness. In its most severe form, slowness of movement can progress to a lack of ability to move at all, called *akinesia.* Although this can be extremely disabling when fully developed, it is one of the symptoms that respond best to the drugs available to treat Parkinson's. Together, rigidity and slowness of movement pose real difficulty.

Body Language, Including Facial Expression

Because of increased rigidity and akinesia, the faces of people who have moderate Parkinson's become somewhat masked and staring, their voices become softer and more monotonous, and the combination of rigidity and bradykinesia makes gesturing more difficult. These symptoms may lead other people to assume that the person who has Parkinson's is unfriendly, uninterested, unintelligent, or even hostile.

At a recent Parkinson's patients' symposium, one gentleman with a masked expression volunteered that he often tells new people he meets, "I look this way because of my Parkinson's disease. I'm actually quite friendly and interested in what you're saying."

Handwriting and Other Hand Dexterity

Together with slowness of movement, rigidity makes it hard for people who have Parkinson's disease to use their fingers and hands to perform fluid motions. As Parkinson's progresses, the process of writing, for example, becomes very slow and handwriting becomes more difficult. A person's handwriting becomes smaller and smaller (called *micrographia*) and sometimes becomes hard to read—a type of communication difficulty (see Chapter 5).

For people who have Parkinson's, rigidity and slowness of movement begin as a very slight problem. The person may feel clumsy buttoning a shirt or trying to write. Slight slowing, awkwardness, or lack of rhythm is also noticed in common repetitive manual tasks such as brushing the teeth, cutting vegetables, or beating eggs.

As time passes, this lack of dexterity increases in severity and intrudes into a person's daily activities. What starts as mild slowness in washing and dressing develops into a significant slowing of movement that requires increasing reliance on others for help with activities such as buttoning, fastening a bra, tying a necktie, washing or combing hair, tying shoelaces, fastening jewelry, applying makeup, rising from a chair, turning over in bed, getting in and out of a car, and using the computer keyboard.

Postural Instability

The *postural reflex*, as we noted in Chapter 3, is a medical description of the many reflexes necessary for people to maintain their balance when standing or walking. *Postural reflex impairment* refers to a loss of function in those reflexes that is typical of Parkinson's disease. Usually the loss first appears when a person has difficulty with walking (gait). Later it may include feeling off balance or falling. Falling is a very difficult symptom to treat in Parkinson's patients, since it often responds poorly to medications, especially later in the disease course. The tendency to fall places a person who has Parkinson's at considerable risk and can significantly interfere with daily activities.

Difficulties with balance may first appear as a feeling of slight unsteadiness when a person turns. In addition, people who have Parkinson's may suddenly find that occasionally they nearly fall down, or do fall down. They are most likely to fall when they turn, walk on an uneven surface, are jostled in a crowd, or arise from sitting in a chair or car or from a crouched position as in gardening.

These falls are particularly disconcerting because they often occur with no warning—no warning sensation of dizziness, lightheadedness, or feeling faint. Because people do not have enough warning to put out their arms for protection, falls can cause injuries such as cuts on the scalp, black eyes, bruises, or even fractures of the wrist and hip (see Chapter 5). Falls can also be triggered by motor block or freezing (see below) and by drops in blood pressure and resulting fainting (see below). It is important to try to differentiate the cause or causes of falls, since different causes may require very different treatment.

Gait Difficulty

Difficulties with walking, like all the other signs of Parkinson's disease, emerge insidiously and gradually. Although initially walking may be quite normal, with time people begin to notice mild alterations. First, a person's arms may not swing quite naturally, or a leg may drag slightly. The previously fluid movements involved in walking may become slightly awkward in an indescribable way (see Chapter 3). As symptoms progress, the person walks more slowly and encounters increasing difficulty keeping up with others. People often comment that they used to be the fastest walker in a group, but now they are the slowest.

As problems with walking become more serious, people who have Parkinson's walk with a kind of shuffle, a short stride in which they do not raise their feet far off the ground. At this stage, they often have difficulty with their balance and may fall. They may feel unsteady on their feet, particularly when they try to turn. If their balance has become significantly impaired, they may fall to the ground with very little apparent reason.

Late in the course of Parkinson's, people may sometimes find their feet suddenly seem glued to the floor and it is extremely difficult to lift them for the next step. This form of sudden arrest of motion is called a *motor block* or *freezing*. Freezing seems to affect walking more than other activities and is especially common when a person first starts to walk, changes direction, turns around including from a standing position such as at the sink in the kitchen or bathroom, or walks through a narrow space, such as a doorway. When people freeze and also have trouble with their balance, they are more likely to fall.

Stooped Posture

People with moderate Parkinson's show a characteristic stooped posture that involves the head, neck, and trunk, all of which lean forward, with the arms held slightly bent at the elbows. Well-meaning family or friends may repeatedly remind the person who has Parkinson's to stand up straight. Although doing so may trigger some limited improvement, the stooping posture returns when the person stops making a special effort to stand up straight.

Although medications for Parkinson's disease may improve posture somewhat, no measure has been successful in preventing the development of this problem.

Nonmotor Symptoms of Moderate Parkinson's Disease

Autonomic System Impairment

The autonomic nervous system manages several body functions, such as digestion, temperature control, gland secretions, and hormones, mostly without our being conscious of its functioning. Parkinson's disease may impair the autonomic nervous system, resulting in a variety of symptoms.

Constipation. Constipation is a common complaint among people who have Parkinson's. It may be something of a nuisance or a more serious problem. People often become concerned about infrequent bowel movements.

First we should note that even in people without Parkinson's disease, constipation is more common as people age. But Parkinson's definitely slows down the gastrointestinal tract from one end to the other, making swallowing, stomach emptying, and movement of the intestines increasingly sluggish. Indeed, constipation may predate the development of other features of Parkinson's by many years. Gastrointestinal motility—movement of material through the intestinal tract—is enhanced by daily exercise, and if people who have Parkinson's become more sedentary because of their walking and balance problems, the problem with slowed intestinal mobility becomes worse. In addition, many medications used to treat the motor symptoms of Parkinson's disease have a slowing effect on the motion of the intestines.

Simple changes in lifestyle and daily routines often can alleviate the problem. Most people who have Parkinson's find they can improve their bowel function by activating the natural reflex to evacuate the bowels in the morning by eating more fiber at breakfast (along with natural bowel stimulants like prunes and coffee), then going for a morning walk at a comfortable pace. They should make sure they drink enough water, at least five to six glasses a day, and increase the roughage (fiber) in their diets. Fiber-rich preparations such as Metamucil or Konsyl (psyllium) can help, along with stool softeners such as Colace (docusate). If these measures do not work, some laxatives are effective. Most importantly, people who have Parkinson's need to watch for regular bowel movements, not frequent ones.

Severe constipation can lead to bowel obstruction, which is a medical emergency. Call or visit your doctor if you are concerned about the absence of regular bowel movements.

Diarrhea. Parkinson's and antiparkinson medications rarely cause diarrhea. For this reason, if you develop diarrhea, you should nearly always assume it is being caused by something other than medications, and your physician should look for other disease processes affecting the bowel. An exception is the COMT inhibitors tolcapone (Tasmar) and entacapone (as Comtan and in Stalevo), which do sometimes cause diarrhea; in its severe form, the diarrhea can be explosive (see Chapters 11 and 13 for more information on COMT inhibitors). Be sure to tell your physician if you have diarrhea while taking tolcapone or entacapone.

One type of diarrhea is a complication of extreme forms of constipation. With severe constipation, stool that remains for some time in the gut can become very hard, dry, and impacted and can almost block the intestine. Liquid stool then flows around the impaction, which leads to a type of diarrhea called *overflow incontinence*. Removal of the impaction will stop the "diarrhea."

Sexual Dysfunction. People who have Parkinson's may find they have difficulty with sexual encounters because their dexterity has decreased, movement is not as spontaneous, changing body position may be more difficult, and tremor increases with excitement. An understanding and reassuring sexual partner can help with some of these difficulties. Remember that the increase in tremor will drop as soon as the excitement level drops and that the increased tremor will do no harm.

Some men with Parkinson's have difficulty achieving and maintaining a sexual erection. The problem may occur in early or moderate Parkinson's, but it is somewhat more likely in advanced stages (see Chapter 5). Prominent very early loss of erectile function might suggest an alternative cause of parkinsonism. Drugs (such as Viagra) that are generally helpful for erectile dysfunction are often also beneficial for men with Parkinson's. Very little study has been done on Parkinson's-related sexual problems in women.

Bladder Dysfunction. A few people who have moderate Parkinson's have difficulty with urination, including the need to urinate very frequently, an urgent need to urinate, or difficulty holding urine, referred to as *urinary incontinence*. Drugs (such as Detrol) that are helpful for "overactive bladder" may be beneficial. Consultation with a urologist may help in identifying other possible contributory factors, such as prostate enlargement in men or bladder prolapse in women. Again, this problem is more likely in advanced disease (see Chapter 5), and when it is prominent in early disease it should raise suspicion of an alternative diagnosis.

Sweating. Unprovoked episodes of excessive sweating are another uncommon symptom. They probably occur because of instability in the autonomic nervous system, which controls temperature regulation. These episodes can be quite dramatic. People report that, regardless of their level of physical activity or the temperature of the environment, they suddenly break out in a drenching sweat. The sweats may last from a few minutes to fifteen or twenty minutes and may be so heavy that people need to change clothes. Occasionally, though not always, a person's skin reddens or flushes.

Excessive sweating is far more likely to occur in people who have more advanced Parkinson's disease and in people who are taking multiple medications for their Parkinson's. Decreasing the amount of carbidopa/levodopa (Sinemet, Madopar) may help alleviate these episodes. Sometimes the sweating occurs exclusively in "off" periods, when the medication level is low (see Chapter 12 for an explanation of "on" and "off" periods). Many people, however, find little correlation between timing of medication and sweating spells. Episodic sweating may appear and then disappear or become markedly better spontaneously, even without adjustments to medications.

Drooling and Swallowing Difficulties

A number of disorders affecting the central nervous system cause drooling, difficulty managing saliva, and problems with swallowing. These problems are rarely encountered early in the course of Parkinson's, but many people who have had the disease for two to four years begin to notice excess saliva in the mouth during the day. This happens because, like other muscular actions, automatic swallowing is simply occurring less frequently, and with the reduction in swallowing, saliva naturally produced in the mouth begins to collect and pool.

People with Parkinson's may wake in the morning with a damp pillow or bedclothes due to pooling of saliva while they sleep, called *nocturnal drooling*. With more advanced Parkinson's disease, drooling during the daytime may appear. Although drooling isn't dangerous, many people are embarrassed by it.

People with this problem routinely carry a tissue or handkerchief in their hand to wipe away excess saliva that appears around their mouth. Trying to suck on a hard candy to stimulate frequent swallowing may be helpful, although some people find this is not a useful therapy because sucking on candy increases the amount of saliva in their mouth. Many of the medications used to treat Parkinson's disease have a tendency to dry the mouth, so the problem of drooling may be addressed this way.

If you experience drooling that is unresponsive to these therapies and is severe, ask your doctor whether treatment with atropine eyedrops under the tongue or with a medication (botulinum toxin) injected into the salivary glands would help you. Another medication that can help alleviate drooling is glycopyrrolate.

For some people, swallowing may become so difficult that they have trouble swallowing pills or they cough or even choke after eating or drinking. If swallowing itself becomes arduous, this creates problems with eating properly, obtaining adequate nutrition, and taking medications. Such problems can lead to weight loss. More seriously, if the swallowing reflex itself is damaged, people can aspirate food particles into their lungs. This is a potentially dangerous problem. Significant problems with swallowing should be reported to the physician (see Chapter 5).

Fortunately, a number of therapies are effective in treating swallowing difficulties at different stages of Parkinson's disease. Speech therapists evaluate the swallowing mechanism, including the function of the mouth, throat, and adjacent structures, and they may recommend changes in food texture or therapies to help with swallowing (see Chapter 5). This symptom may also respond to the medications used to treat Parkinson's motor symptoms.

Disruption of Sleep Patterns

Although no one understands why, Parkinson's is associated with a disruption of sleep patterns. Some people become sleepy during the day, nodding off easily and even falling asleep in social situations and at mealtimes. The problem may be serious enough to be called a *day/night reversal*, in which the person is up at night and asleep during the day.

But even people who sleep well during the night may be excessively drowsy during the day. Their sleepiness may be related to being up at night or to the drugs they are taking. The carbidopa/levodopa and dopamine agonists may be sedating. Rarely, sudden episodes of sleep can occur without warning. More often, there are warning symptoms of drowsiness. These should not be ignored, since falling asleep might occur in situations that could cause harm to the individual and others (e.g., when driving). When antiparkinson medications are the offending agents, this poses a very difficult situation. A person who has Parkinson's requires these medications to avoid stiffness and freezing during the day, yet they may have a sedating effect. Sometimes, but not always, the dosage and scheduling of different drugs can be adjusted to alleviate drowsiness. Unfortunately, the routine use of stimulants, such as amphetamines or methylphenidate (Ritalin), is not often effective in treating this problem, although occasionally people who have excessive daytime sleepiness or drowsiness benefit from low-dose Ritalin (methylphenidate) therapy. Modafinil (Provigil) is another medication that is sometimes helpful to alleviate drowsiness.

When faced with this kind of treatment problem, physicians often do a risk-benefit analysis. For instance, people who do not have true Parkinson's may not be benefiting from the carbidopa/levodopa or dopamine agonists. If the drugs are gradually withdrawn, mental alertness may improve and motor symptoms may not become worse.

Other drugs, such as sleeping pills or drugs used to treat anxiety, depression, muscle spasms, pain, and urinary incontinence, may also contribute to daytime sleepiness. Reducing or eliminating these types of medications may help the person feel more alert.

The most common type of sleep disturbance, known as *sleep fragmentation,* occurs when people wake up several times during the night and have difficulty falling asleep again. Sleep fragmentation may be difficult to treat. Some people wake up because they are uncomfortable, stiff, and unable to turn over in bed or adjust the bedclothes. For some people, their tremor is severe enough in the lighter stages of sleep to waken them and prevent their falling asleep again. The stiffness, immobility, and tremor may be relieved by taking a long-acting Parkinson's medication, such as Sinemet CR, the controlled-release carbidopa/levodopa preparation, at bedtime. Also the use of an extra dose of immediate-release carbidopa/levodopa during the night may help.

Some people have less difficulty falling asleep initially, but wake up frequently and can't get back to sleep. If they are not having difficulty with motor symptoms, they need to look for other causes. Are they drinking too much coffee or other caffeinated beverages? Are they taking selegiline, which can act as a stimulant, in the late afternoon or evening? Are they taking several catnaps during the day and not getting enough exercise? (If so, they may not be fatigued enough to sleep at night.) Keep in mind, too, that even healthy elderly people take more daytime naps and spend fewer hours sleeping at night than younger individuals.

We are reluctant to prescribe sedatives to help people who have Parkinson's fall asleep. They are already taking medications that affect brain function and adding other similar drugs might dull their minds. Sleep medications can have long-lasting effects, and people taking them may experience confusion and disorientation the next day. This is far more frequently a problem with elderly people or people who have preexisting cognitive disturbances.

Changes in lifestyle are the first and best defense against sleep disruption. Most changes are simple: avoid afternoon or evening caffeinated beverages, get more mental and physical exercise, avoid daytime naps and sleeping late in the morning, and try a glass of wine with supper and a bedtime snack such as cookies and warm milk. For some people, a full stomach induces sleep.

Pain

Someone unfamiliar with Parkinson's may regard it as a painless disease, but most people who have longstanding Parkinson's disease would dispute such an assumption. Although pain is less common than more classic symptoms of Parkinson's, many types of pain and sources of discomfort are associated with this disease.

Neck and back pain, frequently radiating to the shoulders or hips, usually is caused by abnormal postures and by decreased flexibility and mobility of the trunk and limbs resulting from rigidity and slowness of movement. One distinctive type of pain associated with Parkinson's is the experience of painful muscle spasms in the foot (see the earlier section on foot cramps). This occurs most often when the person first wakes up in the morning, when antiparkinson medication levels are low. Another type of pain is painful *frozen shoulder*. Frozen shoulder results from lack of spontaneous normal movements, a consequence of slowness of movement (bradykinesia) and rigidity.

The pain attributable to Parkinson's can often be alleviated by taking antiparkinson medications or by increasing or changing the schedule of doses. Sometimes pain is tricky, though. Although initially appearing to be caused by Parkinson's, pain may in fact be due to other causes, such as arthritic changes or muscle spasms that occur in every aging person. It is common for the postural abnormalities and muscle stiffness that occur in Parkinson's disease to aggravate or accentuate these symptoms (e.g., the stooped posture may worsen low back pain caused by degenerative arthritis).

A patient can help his or her physician find the best way to approach the problem by keeping a diary of painful symptoms, recording the day and time when the symptoms occur. For example, if pain commonly occurs when antiparkinson medication levels are low, then an increased dosage or addition of a longer-acting drug may be helpful. Conversely, a few people experience uncomfortable sensations caused by the antiparkinson medication itself, such as scalp burning or headache, and for these individuals an increase in medication is likely to make the problem worse. Physical therapy and a mild exercise program may be helpful. If painful symptoms seem to have no relationship to the timing of antiparkinson medications, a physician may recommend analgesics (pain medications such as ibuprofen, naprosyn, and acetaminophen) to control pain.

Social Isolation and Communication Problems

Although communication problems are not often associated with Parkinson's disease, many of its symptoms disrupt communication on a variety of levels. Most people rely on facial expression and hand gesturing to establish rapport with other people and to add clarity and emphasis to the meaning of their words. A friendly person usually wears a cheerful expression, speaks in a sincere and friendly voice, and uses welcoming gestures. Some of the symptoms of Parkinson's, including loss of facial expression, reduced spontaneous gesturing, and reduced volume of speech (see below), can take those cues away. This may create a socially isolating situation for the person who has Parkinson's disease, who may no longer appear friendly, even when he or she feels friendly.

In addition, some people who have Parkinson's become apathetic, depressed, or anxious. People experiencing such psychological difficulties are often less interested in communicating and socializing and thus become further isolated (see Chapter 6).

Voice

Because of the softening and monotonous nature of the voice in moderate Parkinson's, listeners may have to ask people who have Parkinson's to repeat what they have said. This disease may also cause a slight slurring of speech. Individuals still in the workplace may wish to use a microphone with amplification when making a presentation to a group. They also may want to put special effort into making clear graphs and tables.

Adjustments in medication may sometimes improve a person's speech. In addition, speech therapy designed specifically to meet the needs of people who have Parkinson's, called the Lee Silverman Voice Treatment (LSVT), helps the voice to be stronger and better amplified (see Chapter 14).

People can also supplement their standard methods of communication to keep their lives full and happy. Email, Facebook, and Twitter can be helpful, although bradykinesia and rigidity may interfere with speed and accuracy when using the computer or phone keyboard. Nevertheless, keyboard computer skills are an important new modality that enables many people to remain connected with family, friends, and interests and to keep up-to-date with current events. One patient, in his early nineties, developed such incomprehensible speech that it became impossible for him to communicate by telephone with his children and grandchildren. Email allowed him to reestablish contact with his family.

Skin Rash

For unknown reasons, many people who have Parkinson's develop a particular kind of skin rash, termed *seborrheic dermatitis*. Skin over the scalp and around the facial creases of the nose and mouth may develop an oily, scaly, reddened appearance. The scalp rash responds quite well to tar-based shampoos, and if the rash develops, these shampoos should be used once or twice a week. Facial irritation can be effectively treated by applying mild steroid-based ointments and creams on the affected areas. Care must be taken to avoid getting the cream in the eyes or mouth.

The skin condition is not disabling, but it can be unsightly and annoying. The rash does not respond to medications that are helpful for the motor symptoms of Parkinson's disease.

Inner Restlessness

A sensory phenomenon known as *akathisia* (*a* meaning "not," and *kathisia* referring to sitting) is a sense of inner restlessness, so uncomfortable that the person must get up and walk around to try to relieve the sensation. This sensation is a combination of feelings of unease, discomfort, and unrest. The Yiddish term *shpilkes* is not a bad description for the experience of akathisia.

People with Parkinson's and their families need to be aware of this symptom because it is unusual and is rarely recognized as being related to Parkinson's disease. A person who has never experienced unusual agitation may begin to complain of a sense of unease and restlessness and the feeling of being unable to sit or stand still. Sometimes activity helps people feel better, though sometimes it does not.

People with Parkinson's should discuss any feelings of inner restlessness with their physician. These sensations may be related to the Parkinson's medication and its timing (most often occurring when the medication has worn off; see Chapter 13), or they may be a Parkinson's symptom that will respond to additional medications.

IN THE NEXT CHAPTER we discuss the symptoms of advanced Parkinson's disease. We pause here first to note again that the rate at which people develop Parkinson's symptoms varies greatly. Many people who have Parkinson's who are reading this will never have to cope with many of the symptoms described in this book. We include a discussion of advanced Parkinson's because we are attempting to provide a comprehensive picture of the disease.

CHAPTER 5

Advanced Parkinson's Disease

- *What is advanced Parkinson's disease?*
- *What symptoms are likely to be most serious, and how will they affect the person who has Parkinson's?*
- *Do people die from advanced Parkinson's?*

Parkinson's disease is a progressive disorder: it continues to get worse. For example, as Parkinson's becomes more advanced, people generally have more and more difficulty functioning independently. However, the course of Parkinson's disease varies considerably from person to person. Many people who have Parkinson's never reach an advanced stage, but they live a normal life span and continue to receive significant benefit from their antiparkinson medications. Yet this book would be incomplete if we did not describe advanced Parkinson's disease.

Different people react differently, both physically and emotionally, to Parkinson's disease. People have different levels of *actual* disability, and they also differ in how much a particular symptom may bother them. In addition, some people's bodies respond well to certain medications, while others find they cannot tolerate those medications.

As noted in Chapter 1, it is impossible to predict how any individual's disease will progress. Anything we say on this subject can only be said in very general terms. In general, then, we say that some people who have Parkinson's will advance to significant disability when they have had the disease for nine or ten years, and others may not reach that stage for fifteen years or more. In our experience, those who become significantly disabled in less than five years often have a cause of parkinsonism other than Parkinson's disease (see Chapters 9 and

10). Some people become so disabled that they require skilled nursing home care, but, again, it's almost impossible to predict whether that will happen for any specific individual.

All adults who are competent and able to make decisions about their future health care should create a written document called an *advance directive for health care,* which tells health care professionals what forms of medical care they would accept or would refuse in a specific medical circumstance. All adults should also have a document called a *durable power of attorney for health care,* which designates an individual as the person who will make decisions about their medical care if they become unable to make those decisions themselves. Any adult can have an accident or suddenly become severely ill, and it is better for the individual, the family, and the doctors if these documents have been prepared. People who are diagnosed with Parkinson's disease are no exception. Do not overlook the preparation of these documents, which you can generally create with the help of your state's health department or an attorney.

The life expectancy of people who have Parkinson's disease is only a little shorter than that of people who do not have Parkinson's in the same age group. People usually don't die of Parkinson's, although they may succumb to some of the secondary problems associated with the disease, such as pneumonia or a complication of a fall.

People who had Parkinson's disease thirty or forty years ago faced great difficulties. Today, new medications help people avoid experiencing some of the more severe symptoms once associated with this disease. Research now under way is impressive in its scope and focus and is producing effective new therapies that we hope will, in future, make discussions of advanced Parkinson's unnecessary. With these important caveats, we now give a frank description of the types of problems faced by people who currently have severe, advanced Parkinson's and by their caregivers. Table 5.1 summarizes the problems that are common in advanced stages of the disease.

TREMOR

Tremor may become more severe as Parkinson's disease advances, although a disabling tremor is not very common in the later stages.

TABLE 5.1
PROBLEM AREAS IN ADVANCED PARKINSON'S DISEASE

Cognitive decline and behavioral problems
Communication
Difficulty with urination
Falls
Impaired performance of activities of daily living
Less predictable response to antiparkinson medication
Sexual dysfunction
Swallowing
Walking and balance problems
Weight loss

Many people report that their tremor is not as troubling as it used to be, mainly because of the effectiveness of medications for Parkinson's tremor. For the uncommon situation in which tremor is severe and disabling, the surgical approaches of deep brain stimulation, thalamotomy, or pallidotomy may be considered (see Chapter 16). Such surgery should not be undertaken lightly.

RIGIDITY AND SLOWNESS OF MOVEMENT

As Parkinson's control becomes less reliable, muscle rigidity becomes more severe, and movement becomes extremely slow. Medication helps with many of these symptoms, although the medication plan and dosage often must be repeatedly fine-tuned. Antiparkinson medications continue to be effective in advanced Parkinson's disease, but the response to medications is not as dramatic or as long-lasting as in earlier stages of the disease.

LESS PREDICTABLE RESPONSE TO ANTIPARKINSON MEDICATION

One of the biggest challenges in treating advanced Parkinson's disease is maintaining a steady response to antiparkinson medications. Although Parkinson's symptoms continue to improve or respond to these medications, it is often difficult to achieve a *predictable* response from one dose to the next. As a result, there are periods of the day when motor function is considerably better than at other times. This problem is often called *motor fluctuations*. When motor fluctuations occur, the good periods are commonly referred to as "on" periods and the bad periods as "off" periods. When this problem first begins, the person who has Parkinson's may notice that his or her movement becomes more sluggish and that the limbs feel heavier and fatigued as a medication dose wears off. After several years, the difference in function between the "on" and "off" times tends to become more distinct. The person may be quite functional during "on" time but unable to perform normal activities when "off" time begins (see Chapter 12). The transition between on to off is usually gradual over many minutes, but in some people it can occur quite abruptly, in a matter of seconds. There are many approaches to reducing "off" time. The skills of a neurologist with special expertise in treating Parkinson's disease are important in managing these motor fluctuations.

PAIN

People who have trouble with Parkinson's-related pain are likely to have more problems with this symptom as the disease advances. Three main causes of pain affect people who have Parkinson's.

First, as the disease progresses, the muscles become more rigid, sometimes producing a deep, vague, nagging pain. Such pain is usually alleviated with an adjustment in medication.

Second, changes in muscle tone can result in parkinsonian muscle spasms, or dystonia, which cause a different sort of pain. Frequently these spasms affect the feet, sometimes the hands (see Chapter 4). Often the spasms occur as medication is wearing off, particularly in the morning. The most common solution is to ensure that the level of medication does not become low enough to allow spasm. This can be accomplished by taking a timed-release medication at bedtime or another dose of medication during the night. Occasionally, injections of botulinum toxin into the overactive muscle will weaken it, reduce the spasms, and reduce the accompanying pain.

Third, people who have Parkinson's also get other, more ordinary disorders such as arthritis, bursitis, or tendonitis. The treatments for such problems include pain relievers and are different from treatments for Parkinson's, so the patient and physician need to establish which disorder is causing the difficulty. Sometimes the problem is mixed; people who have Parkinson's may have another cause of pain—for example, sciatica due to a pinched nerve in the back—but this clearly worsens when antiparkinson medications wear off.

Voice

Although speech problems are common in mild to moderate stages of Parkinson's disease, in the advanced stage, communication may be quite significantly impaired. After years with the disease, a person's voice may become progressively softer, more slurred, hesitant, or perhaps excessively fast. Ultimately, others have great difficulty understanding the person's speech. The degree to which speech is impaired often vacillates during the day as the antiparkinson medication cycles between greater and lesser benefit. For some people, speech becomes louder, firmer, and clearer about an hour after a medication dose. For other people, speech may become worse at the peak effect of the medication. They may begin to speak rapidly, with increased slurring. Speech may also become worse as a person becomes tired.

Besides medication, mechanical and electronic aids to communication are also available. A portable microphone helps with soft speech, although it is not likely to be of much use for a person who has significantly slurred speech. There has been some interest in collagen injections into the vocal cords, and for selected patients this approach may improve speech.

More often than other people of the same age, people who have Parkinson's may complain of difficulty finding the word they want. Letter boards or word boards allow the person to point to words that he or she cannot effectively say, and these boards also help those who have difficulty retrieving from their memory bank the word they want. On specially designed keyboards, a particular key produces a programmed message on a computer screen or a message spoken by the computer. One device consists of a computer screen showing numerous little boxes;

each personally programmed box contains a phrase that the patient can point to. Tablet devices, including the iPad, will probably have an important impact on these communication issues in the future.

HANDWRITING

At the more advanced stage of disease, handwriting may become so small and scribbly that it is almost or completely illegible. The process of writing by hand also becomes so slow that it is virtually useless as a convenient means of communication, even if the writing is legible. Handwriting problems are particularly serious when people need to sign checks and other documents.

The degree to which impaired handwriting constitutes a serious disability depends on a number of factors, such as whether people are still in the workplace, whether they live with a caregiver, and whether they can rely on other avenues of communication such as a dictating machine or computer and keyboard or tablet personal computer. For some people this impairment is a serious problem; for others it is just a nuisance.

BALANCE AND MOVEMENT DIFFICULTIES

People who have advanced Parkinson's disease find common physical maneuvers, such as rising to a standing position from a chair or getting in and out of a car, extremely difficult, and they may need to be helped.

Walking difficulty begins as a gait with short steps, progresses to shuffling, and some patients experience being propelled forward (propulsion), sometimes needing an obstruction (e.g., a wall) to stop their forward progress. More common in later disease is freezing, in which the feet seem to be glued to the floor. If moving or turning a corner when the freezing occurs, the person may fall. In fact, balance may become so poor that the person has difficulty maintaining balance while simply standing still. People who have extreme loss of balance may fall with little provocation, or they may even fall spontaneously. These falls may happen so quickly and with so little warning that people have no time to brace their arms for protection, and they often injure themselves. Mild injuries, such as bruises and skin lacerations, are common, but more severe injuries are possible, including head injuries and bone fractures in the hip, arm, wrist, or ribs. Ever-increasing caution and vigilance are required to prevent unnecessary injury. For those who fall frequently, kneepads and elbow pads may be useful.

If falls are not occurring exclusively when medication wears off, they are often very difficult to treat and sometimes are made worse by increasing doses of antiparkinson drugs. When possible we recommend becoming involved in a falls prevention program and working with a physiotherapist for gait retraining. Physiotherapists can teach people who have advanced Parkinson's, as well as their families, new movement strategies to use in rising from a chair or bed, rolling over in bed, and turning around and changing direction while walking. A very common trigger for a fall is when a person pays attention to something in their environment while walking. This may be something as simple as responding to a question or trying to reach out to pick something up. In people who have poor balance and walking impairment, the brain is not capable of handling more than one task efficiently, so it stops paying attention to the walking and concentrates on the second task, with the result that walking deteriorates and a fall may occur. This so-called dual tasking problem is common in later stage Parkinson's disease, and people who have Parkinson's need to learn to attend exclusively to the task of walking and avoid being distracted by their surroundings (obviously, easier said than done).

Because people who have advanced Parkinson's may find it unsafe or perhaps impossible to walk unassisted, they may progress from cane to walker to wheelchair. Many people who have gait problems can improve their balance and walk more freely by simply holding a cane. Some people need a standard walker; others find a walker interferes with their ability to walk. Sometimes people find a four-wheeled rolling walker with handbrakes helpful in maintaining their ability to walk.

A person who has Parkinson's may be reluctant to use a wheelchair, interpreting this as a symbol of the final loss of mobility and independence. Yet this may not be the case. An appropriately used wheelchair allows people who have advanced Parkinson's to get out and socialize and to enjoy shopping, concerts, and shows that might otherwise be too difficult to reach. Use of a wheelchair also protects against injuries, some of which can cause further disability.

SWALLOWING AND DROOLING

Swallowing is something we do without thinking, and when that reflex slows down in Parkinson's disease it causes drooling. Saliva is normally produced all the time and, if not swallowed, it puddles in the mouth. As noted in Chapter 4, drooling usually begins at night, and the person wakes up in the morning to find the pillow or bedsheets wet. Mild, intermittent daytime drooling is common, but only a small number of people who have advanced Parkinson's develop severe problems with drooling.

If drooling is a significant problem, physicians can prescribe anticholinergic drugs such as trihexyphenidyl (Artane), benztropine (Cogentin), and ethopropazine (Parsitan, Parsidol). It is sometimes more convenient and easier to use atropine drops under the tongue once or twice each day to control drooling. The anticholinergics tend to dry the mouth and can often be effective in reducing drooling. These medications can have undesirable side effects, however, such as sleepiness, confusion, or urinary retention. If side effects that affect the brain (such as sleepiness and confusion) are a concern, anticholinergics that work mainly outside the brain—such as oxybutynin (Ditropan) or tolterodine (Detrol)—may be better choices. As noted in Chapter 4, botulinum toxin injections into the salivary glands may be helpful.

Significant swallowing problems do occur, and they may first come to light when people have difficulty swallowing their pills or someone notices they frequently cough, or even choke, during or after eating or drinking. Such problems can cause significant weight loss.

People who have Parkinson's who have these kinds of difficulties with swallowing should immediately alert their physicians because of the danger of aspiration, in which food particles pass into the lungs instead of moving down the esophagus to the stomach. People who aspirate food are at risk of developing *aspiration pneumonia*, an infectious process that makes breathing difficult. If your doctor suspects that your swallowing difficulty poses a risk of aspiration, he or she generally will refer you to a speech pathologist with experience in swallowing dysfunction.

In a common test called a *barium swallow*, the speech pathologist asks the person who has Parkinson's to consume foods and liquids with a variety of textures. The foods and liquids contain barium and are visible on an x-ray as they move through the swallowing process. The radiologist and speech pathologist can carefully observe how swallowing occurs, note any problems, then evaluate the risk of aspiration with different food textures and decide on types of treatments.

The test may show no substantial risk of aspiration, or a substantial risk only under certain circumstances. For example, a person who has Parkinson's may be able to swallow thick, slippery textures well but have difficulty with thin liquids or dry, crumbly foods. The speech pathologist then uses this information to recommend an individual diet.

People who have swallowing problems may need to eat soft foods or food cut into very small pieces. They may also need to drink liquids with thickening agents added or liquid dietary supplements such as Ensure.

For those very few people whose swallowing difficulties and weight loss are not adequately managed with these conservative therapies, a physician can perform a surgical procedure (usually on an outpatient basis) in which a tube is inserted through the abdominal wall into the stomach. The procedure, called a *percutaneous endoscopic gastrostomy* (PEG), is used to provide nutrition and medications to a patient who cannot swallow or for whom the danger of aspiration is too great if he or she swallows food or drink.

The insertion of a PEG tube is a serious step, and people who have Parkinson's and their families should be certain that all less invasive measures, including adjusting the antiparkinson medication, have been exhausted first. The patient's basic quality of life should also be taken into account when considering a PEG. Insertion of a PEG tube allows a person to be fed and to receive proper nutrition, but not all individuals want to take this step. Family members should discuss this among themselves and with the doctor. Another use of a PEG is to administer medications. Rarely patients who have major difficulties swallowing during off episodes benefit from having this access route. We have used this approach very successfully in a small number of patients. Another more common use of a PEG is the application of a continuous form of levodopa treatment, Duodopa, given directly into the small intestine by a pump; Duodopa is available in Scandinavia and Europe and is being investigated in North America currently.

Autonomic System Impairments

Bladder Control and Urinary Difficulties

As noted in Chapter 4, urinary difficulties usually appear as *urinary frequency* (frequent trips to the toilet), *urinary urgency* (a sudden strong urge to urinate immediately), and *urinary incontinence* (loss of urinary control). These difficulties are common complaints, even among people who do not have Parkinson's disease. While it is common for people who have advanced Parkinson's to have urinary difficulties, Parkinson's itself is not always the primary cause. We will first look at urinary problems caused by advanced Parkinson's, then review some other causes of these problems.

If you have any of these problems, you need to discuss them with your doctor—that is the only way he or she can help you. You may find you can be more frank with your doctor if you keep in mind that you are not the only patient with urinary problems; the doctor often helps other people who have these same problems.

A person who has urinary frequency may have to get up two, three, or four times during the night to urinate. This is not normal and it disrupts sleep. Whenever urinary incontinence occurs, a doctor needs to determine whether the person is no longer able to control his or her bladder adequately or whether the main problem is that the person moves so slowly (because of Parkinson's) that he or she cannot get to a toilet in time, especially at night. These two problems must be distinguished, since the approach to treatment is vastly different.

If the problem is true urinary dysfunction, medications can be taken that are helpful in the treatment of urinary frequency, urgency, and incontinence in people who have Parkinson's. Most of these medications are well tolerated. Some medications affect the tone of the bladder and the muscles that control the release of urine; others directly reduce the bladder's irritability and slow down urinary frequency. These drugs include tolterodine (Detrol) and oxybutynin (Ditropan). A bedtime dose of a urinary medication may significantly improve sleep disruption due to bladder complaints, and some new drugs have been introduced to achieve this goal.

When the problem is reaching the bathroom in time, a doctor may alter the basic antiparkinson medications in order to improve the control of slow movement and gait, particularly at night when medication levels tend to be lower. Alternatively, a simple solution might be to keep a urinal or commode near the bed. If people find their episodes of urinary incontinence are unavoidable, they can use incontinence pads. Men may use condom catheters at night or even during the day. The condom catheter fits over the penis like a condom and has a tube at the end to collect and drain the urine into a bag. No tubes are inserted into the penis.

A number of common urinary problems are unrelated to Parkinson's disease. Urinary tract infections (UTIs), for example, produce symptoms identical to urinary problems due to Parkinson's, although UTIs may also cause fever and pain on passing urine. When a person who has Parkinson's disease develops urinary frequency and urgency, the physician needs to first rule out a UTI as the cause of these symptoms, even when the person does not have a fever or any pain when urinating. Such infections can be detected with a simple analysis of the urine, and they are easy to treat with oral antibiotics. Most people who have advanced Parkinson's who develop urinary frequency and urgency have no sign of infection. Alternatively, some elderly patients with Parkinson's disease may experience confusion as the only feature of a urinary tract infection, so it is important to consider and exclude this possible explanation when a patient's mental state changes for no apparent reason.

The most common cause of urinary frequency and urgency in men in their sixties and seventies is *benign prostatic hypertrophy,* or enlargement of the prostate gland. The prostate gland encircles the urethra, a tube that carries the urine out of the body. If the prostate enlarges, it squeezes the urethra and causes urinary difficulties.

Men with Parkinson's who develop urinary symptoms must be evaluated by a urologist who has experience with the urinary problems seen in Parkinson's disease. An experienced urologist can help the neurologist determine whether the degree of prostate enlargement appears consistent with the severity of the urinary symptoms. Prostate surgery to reduce the size of the prostate makes sense only if the urologist is relatively certain that the prostate size, not the Parkinson's disease, is the main culprit. The urologist may perform special tests to measure bladder function, including a cystoscopy, which involves putting a tube up the urethra into the bladder. If Parkinson's is the major source of the symptoms, prostate surgery may actually worsen rather than improve the symptoms.

When women with Parkinson's disease have urinary problems, they need to be evaluated by both a gynecologist and a urologist. Childbirth may cause the muscles surrounding the pelvic organs to be lax, and this sometimes causes women to have urinary frequency, urgency, and incontinence later in life. Some women require surgery to reposition a bladder that has dropped lower into the pelvic area.

Constipation

Constipation is a very common problem in advanced Parkinson's disease, and it becomes more severe as the disease progresses. For some people who have Parkinson's, constipation is a very disruptive problem. For more information, including therapies, see Chapter 4.

Sexual Dysfunction

Some people who have Parkinson's experience sexual dysfunction, but many do not. The most common sexual problem for men is failure to achieve an erection. Erectile dysfunction (impotence) may occur at any stage of Parkinson's, but it becomes somewhat more likely (although not a certainty) during the advanced stage. It can be associated with Parkinson's itself, but many other disorders, including diabetes and vascular disease, can cause this problem or make it worse.

Many treatments are available for this type of sexual dysfunction. Remedies that work reasonably well include sildenafil (Viagra) or tadalafil (Cialis), taken as an orally administered pill, or alprostadil (Caverject), a painless self-administered injection of medication into the penis. Some mechanical devices, such as a vacuum pump, are also available to assist an erection. Surgical procedures are also available but are rarely helpful for men with Parkinson's. Some men who have Parkinson's disease develop an increased interest in sex as a side effect of antiparkinson medications. In some this becomes excessive and can have negative effects on the relationship with their partner. This can be further complicated if the man has erectile dysfunction. It is important to have a frank and open discussion about these issues with your doctor rather than hiding what can sometimes be a significant and damaging problem.

Sexual dysfunction in women with Parkinson's disease has not been well studied. Preliminary studies suggest that women may experience less sexual satisfaction and difficulty achieving orgasm, but further studies are needed.

A warm and loving relationship between partners is surely an advantage in dealing with any chronic illness, including Parkinson's disease. Lucille Carlton's book *In Sickness and in Health: Sex, Love, and Chronic Illness* discusses many ways (physical and emotional) of showing love even when physical problems prevent sexual intercourse. (This book is out of print. You can look for it in used-book stores, or a company that searches for out-of-print books [a number of these companies are found on the Internet] may be able to locate a copy for you.)

Orthostatic Hypotension, or Fainting after Rising

Normally, when we stand from a seated or supine position, our autonomic nervous system rapidly readjusts our blood pressure in order to maintain a smooth and uninterrupted blood flow to our brain. In a number of neurodegenerative disorders such as Parkinson's disease and multiple system atrophy (MSA), this reflex becomes sluggish. Medications used to treat Parkinson's disease can accentuate this problem. On standing up, especially after being seated for a long time, an individual becomes dizzy or lightheaded for a few moments until the blood pressure and blood flow to the brain readjust. Another symptom of this problem may be fainting on standing or achiness across the shoulders. This condition is called *orthostatic hypotension*. (Hypotension is low blood pressure; hypertension is high blood pressure.)

There are several approaches to this problem. Most obviously, rising more slowly and standing still to "get one's bearings" before beginning to walk can be helpful. For people who have orthostatic hypotension, fluid pools in the legs while they are sitting down, and wearing supportive elastic stockings can help reduce the amount of fluid.

Medications available to treat orthostatic hypotension include fludrocortisone (Florinef) and midodrine (ProAmatine). Other strategies include increasing the total blood volume, which aids in maintaining blood pressure at a somewhat higher level. It is important to take in enough fluid, at least six eight-ounce glasses a day, especially in hot weather, and preferably water. Some drinks, such as tea, coffee, and some sodas, may act as diuretics and remove some of the fluids from the body, so if you drink them, drink water as well. A higher salt intake also traps more fluids and helps maintain fluid volume. People can use the saltshaker more liberally, drink bouillon, or take salt (NaCl) tablets. Elevating the head of the bed by placing the head-end legs on six-inch blocks can improve orthostatic hypotension. This effect is not obtained by bending the head end up from the middle as in the standard hospital-type bed.

Some medications that decrease high blood pressure can accentuate orthostatic hypotension. Some (e.g., "water" pills or diuretics) work by making the body excrete more fluid, and some directly relax blood vessels. A physician may need to reevaluate the use of these medications for people who have orthostatic hypotension and allow somewhat higher blood pressures in order to avoid this excessive drop in blood pressure when changing position.

DRUG-INDUCED SYMPTOMS

Antiparkinson medications can cause drug-related side effects, such as stomach upset, nausea, dizziness, fatigue, orthostatic hypotension (see above), drug-related motor fluctuations, dyskinesia, and hallucinations (see Chapter 12). *Side effects* are not signs of drug toxicity but unintended consequences that may emerge when taking certain medications. Side effects of medications are usually undesirable, such as a rash when taking an antibiotic or sleepiness when taking an antihistamine. Sometimes side effects come in handy; for example, the dry mouth that results from some Parkinson's medications can be useful for controlling drooling. And some side effects are intolerable, such as insomnia caused by some antibiotics. For the most part, when a medication is discontinued, the side effects come to an end, although some may take time to disappear completely.

Toxic effects are different. When a drug is toxic it causes long-term harm. There is no evidence that Parkinson's drugs are toxic.

Specific information on the side effects of medications is included in the discussions of those medications in Chapters 12 and 13. In general, because levodopa and its related medications are so widely and effectively used for treatment of Parkinson's, they are also responsible for many of the side effects experienced by people who have Parkinson's disease. The amount of medication, the types of drugs, or the schedule on which they are taken may need to be adjusted to eliminate side effects. Be sure to tell your doctor if you are having difficulties you believe are caused by your medications.

BEHAVIORAL PROBLEMS AND PSYCHIATRIC SYMPTOMS

The behavioral and psychiatric symptoms of advanced Parkinson's fall into two categories: those caused by the disease and those that result from medication (having the disease can also make a person more likely to have certain medication-induced behavioral side effects). As noted above, Chapter 12 discusses drug-related symptoms in detail. Here we mainly discuss symptoms caused by the disease.

Symptoms Caused by Parkinson's

Decline in Mental Abilities. For most of the course of their disease, people who have Parkinson's maintain good cognitive function. But after five, ten, or more years, in advanced disease, confusion and memory problems, known as *dementia,* may develop. One in every four or five people who have Parkinson's will have dementia severe enough to interfere with daily functioning, and after fifteen years of Parkinson's more than half of all people will have this problem (see Chapter 6).

Depression and Anxiety. A significant number of people who have Parkinson's suffer from depression or anxiety, or both. Depression brings feelings of diminished self-worth and hopelessness, disrupted sleep,

and appetite changes. Anxiety also causes feelings of discomfort ranging from mild to severe. The standard medical treatments for depression and anxiety have been successful for people who have Parkinson's
(see Chapters 3, 6, and 13).

Fatigue. People who have Parkinson's who tire easily, far out of proportion to the effort they have expended, need to know that they are
not alone. An estimated 40 percent of people who have Parkinson's
have some fatigue disability, and it may be severe. Fatigue is also very
common in a number of brain diseases, including other neurodegener-
ations and multiple sclerosis. Fatigue often triggers a vicious cycle in
which the person is less and less active, resulting in further reduction
of stamina. Although it may sound paradoxical, an increase in activity and exercise may help increase strength and endurance. Currently
available medications are not very effective in treating fatigue.

Drug-Induced Symptoms

Because the medications used to alleviate Parkinson's symptoms
work by affecting brain chemistry, they are sometimes associated with
undesirable psychiatric and behavioral side effects. As Parkinson's becomes more advanced, higher doses of drugs are required and side
effects become more of a problem. Particularly troubling side effects
are drug-related hallucinations and delusions (false beliefs). These side
effects do not occur in every patient, but when they do occur they may
be very distressing to the person who has Parkinson's and his or her
family members.

When the dosage of the drug causing side effects is reduced or the
drug is stopped, these alarming mental side effects disappear, but the
motor symptoms return. In other words, the problem faced by patient
and doctor may be a choice between drug-induced hallucinations and
severe tremor or slowness. The choice is not necessarily this stark,
however. A number of new drugs and new combinations of old drugs
are now available that can reduce psychiatric symptoms and permit
the person to continue receiving the benefits of antiparkinson medication. In advanced disease, many people end up taking multiple drugs; a
careful review of medications with your doctor may lead to the discontinuation of many medications without worsening of the symptoms of
Parkinson's—and with improvement in cognition.

WEIGHT LOSS OF UNKNOWN CAUSE

Weight loss for no obvious reason may occur in individuals with advanced Parkinson's disease, even when swallowing is not a problem. The patient is usually referred to her or his primary care physician for a thorough general medical examination to search for other medical conditions that may be causing the weight loss. Often this evaluation does not reveal any other cause. Although the precise cause remains unclear, we assume that this sort of weight loss is related to the advanced Parkinson's symptoms themselves.

PROBLEMS OF DAILY LIVING

In advanced Parkinson's disease, the routine activities of dressing, hygiene, and feeding become increasingly slow and ponderous. Family members may find they increasingly need to assist with daily activities such as fastening buttons, snaps, and zippers, or putting on shirts, pants, and undergarments.

Occupational therapists can show patients and families a variety of ways for dealing with loss of dexterity and slowness. Their catalog of devices that can assist people who have Parkinson's includes hook-and-loop closures (such as Velcro) on shoes and clothing, long shoehorns, and eating utensils that are easier to manipulate. The home can be made more convenient and safer with bathroom grab bars, shower seats, elevated toilet seats, and bedside commodes. These devices do more than just help people who have Parkinson's carry out simple tasks; they enable them to remain independent. Such independence is extremely important for people who have Parkinson's, for both physical and psychological reasons.

NEW THERAPIES for people who have Parkinson's disease are being developed all the time, and we hope that in the coming years they will make this description of severe, advanced illness a record of only historical interest.

CHAPTER 6

Behavioral Changes and Psychiatric Symptoms

- *How are mental abilities and memory affected by Parkinson's disease?*
- *What about mood and motivation?*
- *What psychiatric symptoms may develop as a side effect of taking antiparkinson medications?*

The characteristic TRAP symptoms of Parkinson's disease—tremor, rigidity, slowness of movement, and difficulties with balance or posture—all involve motor function. But Parkinson's is generally a much more complicated, multifaceted disorder. It can cause a wide range of cognitive, behavioral, and psychiatric symptoms, and so can the drugs used to treat it. In this chapter we discuss these symptoms and what can be done to manage them.

COGNITIVE SYMPTOMS

In early Parkinson's disease, people seldom experience a significant alteration in their ability to think and communicate. Because their cognitive (mental) abilities are intact, they do not experience difficulty carrying out any mental aspects of their job responsibilities. In fact, early cognitive problems usually point to a form of parkinsonism other than true Parkinson's disease (see Chapters 9 and 10).

This does not mean, however, that people who have early and moderate Parkinson's disease have no alterations in their cognitive functions. Formal neuropsychological testing is not routine or required in the treatment of Parkinson's, but people who have Parkinson's who do undergo such testing often demonstrate a variety of minor abnormalities when compared with age-matched people who do not have Parkinson's disease. Testing involves the administration of a series of questionnaires under the guidance of a neuropsychologist to evaluate abilities in areas such as memory, problem solving, puzzle solving, reading comprehension, abstract thinking, insight, and judgment. For individuals with Parkinson's disease, these tests generally show evidence of some specific and mild cognitive changes. Most people can compensate for these specific changes, so their performance on the job and in their home life is not seriously disrupted.

In some settings, neuropsychological testing in early Parkinson's disease can be helpful as a diagnostic tool. When people who have early Parkinson's demonstrate the typical and expected deficiencies associated with the disorder at this stage, the neurologist can be reassured that the diagnosis is correct. If in formal neuropsychological testing a person exhibits more serious cognitive or personality changes early in the disease, then a different neurologic disorder, perhaps one that affects more areas of the brain than does Parkinson's, needs to be considered. These kinds of neurologic disorders may be caused by a form of parkinsonism called *dementia with Lewy bodies* (or *diffuse Lewy body disease*), or even by Alzheimer's disease (see Chapter 10). An accurate diagnosis of neurologic disorders allows individuals and their families to plan appropriately for the future, with an understanding of how the disease is likely to affect them as time goes by.

There has been considerable interest in the idea that the findings of early neuropsychological testing may determine which people who have Parkinson's disease are at greater risk of later developing more significant cognitive problems. But proving or disproving this idea would require long-term follow-up of patients, and unfortunately, adequate studies have not been done. At this time, therefore, the results of early neuropsychological tests in patients who have no evidence of cognitive dysfunction cannot be used to predict whether or not a person who has Parkinson's disease will eventually develop serious cognitive problems.

In the later stages of Parkinson's, more profound memory loss and confusion may develop. Approximately 20 to 25 percent of people in the advanced stages of the illness develop *dementia,* and in the very advanced stage of Parkinson's (longer than fifteen to twenty years) more than 50 percent of people develop dementia, the medical term used to describe thinking and memory problems severe enough to interfere with day-to-day functioning. We cannot predict which people who have Parkinson's disease will develop this disabling problem.

Reduction or withdrawal of some of the antiparkinson medication may occasionally result in improvement in a person's mental state. New medications can provide some help with memory problems (see Chapter 13). Promising new avenues of treatment are also being actively explored, including drugs that were originally developed and marketed for use in Alzheimer's disease.

BEHAVIORAL SYMPTOMS

As noted in Chapter 3, people who have Parkinson's may experience behavioral changes such as depression, anxiety, apathy, and fatigue. For a small percentage of people, these are the initial symptoms of very early Parkinson's, although these symptoms are so vague that physicians are unlikely to link them with the onset of Parkinson's disease. We occasionally see patients who were initially treated for depression then were later found to have emerging Parkinson's disease.

Behavioral symptoms like depression, anxiety, fatigue, or apathy may occur in isolation or together as "comorbid conditions." For example, depression and anxiety commonly occur together. Similarly, depression and apathy or depression and fatigue may be present at the same time. Fortunately, many medications that reduce depression also reduce anxiety. There are no medicines specifically approved to treat apathy, and apathy can be difficult to treat. In some cases, better treatment of the Parkinson's symptoms themselves, or relief of depression, results in less apathy. At times, behavioral symptoms and Parkinson's symptoms can create a "vicious cycle" where the Parkinson's symptoms are troubling, resulting in greater anxiety and depression—and this increase in emotional symptoms results in greater difficulty with coping and adjusting to the Parkinson's symptoms. This difficult cycle may be broken by treating each of the component parts: the Parkinson's symptoms, depression, or anxiety. Nonpharmacologic approaches like exercise or greater social activity may also relieve behavioral symptoms.

Depression

Depression is a significant problem in about 40 percent of people who have Parkinson's. As noted in Chapter 3, severe depression is different from the dismay and grief people experience when they find out they have a degenerative neurologic illness. Many people who have Parkinson's are also demoralized and frustrated with a body that no longer responds as it once did. In fact, mild but pervasive depression is very common in Parkinson's, and more research attention is being directed at this problem. But severe depression typically involves unstoppable feelings of hopelessness, helplessness, and diminished self-worth, as well as disruption of appetite and sleep.

Some physicians believe that severe depression in people who have Parkinson's results from disruption of neurotransmitter systems in the brain. There is some evidence for this. For example, many people who have Parkinson's experience depression before they have any other signs of Parkinson's. This suggests that at least some forms of depression may reflect underlying changes in brain chemistry. Also, if depression were solely a personal reaction to disability, we would expect it to increase at the same rate as the disease advances, but studies have not been able to confirm this.

We believe depression in Parkinson's is largely due to changes in the neurochemistry of the brain. Dismay over having a chronic progressive disease contributes to depression, but biochemical changes play a large role in the development of severe depression in Parkinson's disease.

Physicians may overlook the early symptoms of Parkinson's disease when depression appears early in the disorder, because of the considerable overlap between the symptoms of Parkinson's and the symptoms of depression. People who are depressed may appear to have symptoms of Parkinson's, and people who have Parkinson's have symptoms that mimic depression. For example, the loss of facial expression—the masked face—may be mistaken for a depressed appearance, and the slowness and stooped posture of people who have Parkinson's may be mistaken for the gait and posture of a person who has depression. When people who have Parkinson's are mistakenly diagnosed with having only depression, the correct diagnosis will become evident with time as the typical resting tremor appears or as slowness begins to interfere with independent daily functioning.

Depression can be successfully treated with a wide range of antidepressant medications (see Chapter 13). A physician takes into account a person's full medical history and current symptom profile and then recommends specific antidepressant medications. To give the antidepressant an adequate trial, a person usually should take it in adequate doses for a month or two. If it is not effective or causes unwanted side effects, another antidepressant should be tried. Severe depression may rarely require more intensive psychiatric care or hospitalization.

Anxiety

About 40 percent of people who have Parkinson's also suffer from anxiety, or nervousness and agitation. Anxiety may occur in conjunction with depression or it may appear on its own. Anxiety can cause considerable disability, but people may be reluctant to acknowledge anxiety as a problem, even when it causes serious disruptions in their lives. In the same way that the slowness of Parkinson's disease can be confused with depression, the Parkinson's tremor can be confused with anxiety.

As noted in Chapter 3, people experiencing significant anxiety may have difficulty with both job performance and socialization. Anxiety may interfere with their ability to speak in front of a group of people, or it may turn a pleasant social gathering into a disturbing experience. Salespeople may report that their anxiety makes them less effective with customers. And some people avoid social settings to avoid feeling the discomfort of their anxiety. As Parkinson's progresses, many people find they become anxious in situations that earlier would not have caused such stress or anxiety. They become apprehensive when they drive in busy traffic or answer an unexpected ringing of the doorbell. At its most extreme, anxiety can produce debilitating episodes called *panic attacks*.

A variety of medications, including the selective serotonin reuptake inhibitors (SSRIs) (see Chapter 13), have helped many people successfully overcome their feelings of anxiety. Symptoms of anxiety are sometimes related to an underlying depression, so-called *agitated depression,* which requires specific treatment. Some people are reluctant to take medication for anxiety, and they are often surprised by how helpful these drugs can be. As one person who has Parkinson's said, "I still have the same thoughts as before, but they just don't bother me like they used to." You should talk to your doctor about medication for anxiety or depression if Parkinson's symptoms interfere with your daily function or quality of life, including socialization, recreation, and employment.

Apathy and Amotivation

Apathy and *amotivation* refer to a state in which a person loses his or her interest in all sorts of activities that were previously a source of gratification and enjoyment. The person's career, hobbies, and socializing may all seem less stimulating and satisfying than they used to be. Apathy can be an extremely disabling symptom, robbing an individual of the motivation to engage in new and productive activities. Nonetheless, doctors often do not recognize that apathy is part of Parkinson's disease. Apathy may be a significant problem at any stage of Parkinson's. It may be associated with depression or dementia, but frequently amotivation is an isolated behavioral symptom in people who have Parkinson's.

The spouse of a person who has Parkinson's disease is often the one who reports that the person seems less and less interested in her or his usual activities. Some people lose interest in pursuing new interests or participating in social activities outside the home, such as going to a play or concert or visiting with friends and relatives. They may also lose interest in old hobbies and show little initiative to make plans. And they may become increasingly withdrawn and less likely to participate in conversation. Apathy can also interfere with a person's ability and energy to cope with the changing circumstances of his or her life related to the symptoms of Parkinson's disease.

There is increasing interest in the relationship between the neurotransmitter dopamine and the loss of motivation and initiative. Research is under way to identify medication that will help people who have motivational disorders. The currently available medications have variable effectiveness.

Fatigue

Again, about 40 percent of people who have Parkinson's report feeling fatigued out of proportion to any effort they have expended. Fatigue can occur at any stage of the disease—early, moderate, or advanced—but doctors often overlook this as part of Parkinson's disease. Nor, unfortunately, do doctors understand the causes of fatigue.

Fatigue can be disabling, although its effects vary widely. The term is generally used to refer to a sense of exhaustion or tiredness but not true sleepiness (although the two complaints can coexist). This can be confused with true excessive daytime sleepiness where people report feeling sleepy with dozing off and feel a need for naps in the daytime. Alternatively, it can be confused with the slowness and heaviness of the limbs in Parkinson's disease as a sensation of loss of energy. Some people report that their fatigue is relieved when they take their anti-parkinson medications, while others report exactly the opposite, with greater fatigue as well as the experience that their medications make them feel sleepy.

Fatigue may occur with or without depression and amotivation, and it is often challenging for a physician to discriminate among these symptoms. Medications are available for depression and anxiety, but both amotivation and fatigue are considerably more difficult to treat with currently available drugs. Treating a patient for depression or anxiety sometimes helps both the patient and the doctor understand exactly what the underlying problem is—depression and anxiety, or apathy, or fatigue.

DRUG-INDUCED BEHAVIORAL AND PSYCHIATRIC SYMPTOMS

The drugs used to treat Parkinson's are designed to affect brain chemistry (see Chapter 11). As a result, they can also produce behavioral changes and psychiatric symptoms such as vivid dreams, nightmares, nonthreatening visual hallucinations, delusions (false beliefs), paranoia, disorientation, and impulse control disorders (for example, hypersexuality, pathological gambling, obsessive shopping or eating).

Drug-induced psychiatric disorders are rare in early Parkinson's, but they become more common as the disease progresses. People who are elderly are at increased risk for drug-induced behavioral and psychiatric problems. People who have more advanced Parkinson's have taken the drugs for a longer time, and they need higher dosages of drugs and multiple drugs used in combination. All drugs used to treat Parkinson's disease can produce behavioral changes or psychiatric symptoms. If drug-induced psychiatric symptoms appear in a patient being treated for Parkinson's, the symptoms will resolve entirely if the drug causing the symptoms is discontinued. Unfortunately, discontinuing antiparkinson drugs can result in unacceptably increased motor symptoms. Yet, reducing the dosage of the drugs or changing medications is often helpful. In some situations, medications that specifically treat the psychiatric symptoms are needed. Because of the risk of psychiatric symptoms, Parkinson's medications should be started at a low dose, then slowly increased under careful monitoring.

Although it only rarely happens, families and caregivers need to know that in extreme cases of drug-induced behavioral alterations, an individual may become severely agitated and very difficult to control. This can be a medical emergency, requiring admission to the hospital so that the person will be in a safe environment while medications are readjusted.

Vivid Dreams

People who have Parkinson's sometimes develop vivid dreams and nightmares. Both may have a very realistic quality to them, and the nightmares may be quite frightening. These dreams and nightmares may be so vivid that people confuse what is real and what is a dream. Sometimes people have difficulty distinguishing between dreams while asleep and hallucinations while awake. Nightmares may be accompanied by violent thrashing movements. Vivid dreams may also be accompanied by talking or screaming out loud. This acting out or responding to a dream by shouting or moving about is known as a *REM* (for *r*apid *e*ye *m*ovement) *behavioral disorder.* It can become so disruptive that the bed partner has to move to another bed or room to sleep.

REM behavioral disorder is recognized as a common problem in Parkinson's disease, as well as in some other neurodegenerative diseases. This disorder may even precede the development of other symptoms and the diagnosis of Parkinson's by several years, so, clearly, antiparkinson medication alone is not causing the problem. Late in the disease, if nighttime disruptions become frequent, the doctor may need to reduce or eliminate nighttime antiparkinson medication. If that fails to relieve the problem, the doctor may need to consider also reducing the overall dosage of antiparkinson medications during the day. The use of low dose clonazepam or melatonin at bedtime can be extremely useful to treat REM behavioral disorder.

Visual Hallucinations

Hallucinations are perceptions that an object, person, place, or thing is present when in reality it is not. Visual hallucinations, both non-threatening (benign) and threatening, are much more common in people who have Parkinson's than are auditory hallucinations (hearing voices or music) or tactile hallucinations (feeling sensations on the skin).

Persons with advanced Parkinson's who have been taking antiparkinson medications for many years often begin to have nonthreatening visual hallucinations. For example, a pillow on a couch may be seen as a person's head, or a tree in the back yard may be transformed into a person or a group of children. Another type of "almost" hallucination is the "sense of a presence" over the person's shoulder or perceived in their peripheral vision. This is not actually a formed perception but a "sense" of one.

Some people understand they are having visual hallucinations and may not be upset by them; others have difficulty discriminating what is real and what is not and may become alarmed by their hallucinations. For example, a woman sitting in her living room in the evening might become anxious if she sees a strange man walking in the house or looking through the window. People sometimes describe seeing family members (often their parents) who died long ago in their house with them, or they see small elflike children, pets, or insects that are not real.

When people with Parkinson's who experience hallucinations are unable to discriminate reality from hallucination, they may, understandably, become disturbed and agitated, and this disorientation may make them difficult to care for. Some people, though, understand fully that the "dog following them around" or the "group of people" in the apartment are not real, and they are curiously undisturbed by their hallucinations. Family members are often startled to hear their relative with Parkinson's describe these experiences when a doctor takes a medical history, since the family has rarely, if ever, heard the person mention them. An individual who has infrequent visual hallucinations that produce no particular consequences may not require treatment. The physician needs to exercise caution when adding new antiparkinson medications that are likely to make the problem worse.

Delusions

People who have advanced Parkinson's disease who have been taking antiparkinson medications for many years may experience delusions (false beliefs). Delusions may take the form of believing a spouse is having an affair or thinking money has been stolen. A person who has delusions may also feel unfairly persecuted and experience what are called *paranoid delusions*.

Although most people who have Parkinson's disease do not become so delusional or dissociated that they require residential care, some patients with advanced Parkinson's do require full-time skilled nursing care. One study evaluating why patients with severe, advanced Parkinson's disease are admitted to nursing homes found the most common reason was hallucinations and their associated behavioral problems.

Fortunately, we can take steps to deal with this complex set of problems. First, hallucinations and delusions may be eliminated or reduced in severity by changing, reducing, or eliminating antiparkinson medications. If antiparkinson medications can't be eliminated, a number of drugs are available for treating delusions.

The Dopamine Dysregulation Syndrome, Punding and Impulse Control Disorders

A small proportion of people taking antiparkinson medication develop a variety of symptoms that have been lumped under the term *dopamine dysregulation syndrome* (DDS). These symptoms include aggressive, agitated and grandiose behavior, hoarding of antiparkinson medications, and taking more than is needed to maintain mobility (often with the result of marked levodopa-induced dyskinesias). This is thought to be a drug-addiction related disorder and, as in other drug addictions, patients typically deny their problem and hide the truth about how much and how often they are taking their medication. The DDS usually occurs in young men taking excessive doses of levodopa/carbidopa. Some patients demonstrate repetitive obsessive performance of sometimes purposeless activities such as collecting, sorting, or itemizing (called "punding"). Punding describes aimless stereotyped behaviors performed for long periods at the expense of other activities and can including behaviors such as taking apart and assembling mechanical objects such as clocks, arranging and rearranging stamp collections, continuously brushing hair, incessantly sorting through handbags or even taking repetitive meaningless walks in the neighborhood.

Impulse control disorders (ICD) are now recognized as a complication of the use of the dopaminergic drugs used to treat Parkinson's. Most commonly, the dopamine agonists (ropinirole, pramipexole) are implicated, but LD/CD (Sinemet) can play a role. Recent studies indicate that if thoroughly searched for, as many as 15 percent of patients with Parkinson's taking dopaminergic drugs may exhibit one of these ICDs. ICDs are characterized by pathological gambling, excessive or abnormal sexual interests, compulsive shopping, excessive eating, and unusual and repetitive use of the Internet and computer. People who have ICDs are likely to be younger, have a smoking or alcohol history, have a family history of gambling disorders, be single, and live in the United States. People who have Parkinson's and ICD have more functional impairment in activities of daily living, and therefore it is important to recognize this problem. The symptoms may be isolated (e.g., gambling) or may occur in multiple combinations. Examples include a person with no prior interest in pornography or history of gambling that over a period of weeks to months spends hours per day watching pornography or begins to lose thousands of dollars per week at a casino. Other examples include a wealthy individual who feels compelled to buy expensive jewelry even though he has no need or use for it, to the point that he must hide the purchases from his family. These problems are largely taken care of by reducing or eliminating the causative drugs, under the supervision of a physician. Keep in mind that gambling addiction is a widespread problem in modern society, and when it occurs in someone with Parkinson's disease it may or may not be a complication of antiparkinson medication.

How Do Antiparkinson Drugs Cause Behavioral and Psychiatric Symptoms?

Psychological and behavioral symptoms are induced by medications that act on the dopamine system. Dopamine is key to more than one system in the brain: it is crucial to the systems that fundamentally control motor behavior and to the systems involved in emotional responses (particularly responses to reward), mood, and behavior. Thus the medications designed to act on the dopamine motor systems also influence the emotional/mood/behavior systems.

The sometimes frightening symptoms described above are generally signs of dopamine overstimulation in the emotional/mood/behavior systems. This does not involve an overdose in the usual sense—in which a patient has accidentally taken too much medication or a doctor has overprescribed medication. Rather, over many years of taking dopamine medications, a hypersensitivity emerges in the dopamine system. People who have had Parkinson's for some time may develop these behavioral abnormalities even though they are taking the same dosage of medication they have taken for many years.

Sometimes a small change, such as a slight increase in dosage or the introduction of a new drug (such as a single sleeping pill), triggers the emergence of the symptoms. Any of these psychiatric symptoms may also be induced or worsened following an operation such as hip surgery or by an infection such as bladder infection or pneumonia. Finally, as mentioned earlier, a small proportion of people abuse their antiparkinson medication and develop psychiatric side effects as a consequence of this addictive behavior.

SIDE EFFECTS VERSUS THE DESIRED EFFECTS OF THE MEDICATION

For many people who have Parkinson's, the behavioral and psychiatric symptoms markedly diminish, if not completely disappear, if their medication dosage is reduced. Many people take several medications at once: perhaps levodopa to increase the amount of dopamine in the brain, another drug to enhance the levodopa, and medications for depression or anxiety. A physician may have a difficult time determining which of these medications is causing a side effect. Sometimes, no one drug is at fault, and the problem is caused by a combination of several drugs that multiplies their effect—often called the *synergistic* effect. Side effects can be diminished by decreasing the number of drugs and simplifying the medication schedule.

The real problem is that people may require high dosages to control their motor symptoms—tremor, rigidity, slowness, and balance problems—and these dosages may be above the threshold that causes their delusions and hallucinations. For example, consider a person with levodopa-induced hallucinations whose hallucinations can be eliminated by reducing the levodopa dosage, but when the levodopa dosage is reduced, the person is unable to walk independently. Such a person might be helped by different medication, or current medications may need to be readjusted to produce the greatest benefit with the least side effects. These problems must be managed on an individual basis by the physician.

Drugs That May Contribute to Behavioral and Psychiatric Symptoms

Anticholinergics. The anticholinergic family of drugs exert most of their effect on the nerve cells that use *acetylcholine* as their neurotransmitter. Tremor may be reduced by balancing the effects of the acetylcholine neurotransmitter system with the dopamine neurotransmitter system, because the two systems interact (see Chapter 11). Anticholinergic medications may be used to restore a semblance of balance between these two systems. These drugs, used mainly to control Parkinson's tremor, include trihexyphenidyl (Artane), benztropine (Cogentin), procyclidine (Kemadrin), and ethopropazine (Parsitan, Parsidol). Especially in elderly people, they may produce confusion and forgetfulness, and they may also contribute to the development of hallucinations and delusions. (See Chapter 13 for more information on anticholinergics.)

For a variety of reasons, elderly people often are more sensitive to drugs than younger people, and anticholinergic drugs are particularly problematic. They need to be used with caution and in the lowest effective dosage.

If you are taking anticholinergic medication, you may want to check with your doctor to find out whether he or she started you with the lowest possible dose.

Drugs Affecting the Dopamine System. The drugs that affect the dopamine system, including carbidopa/levodopa (Sinemet, Atamet), carbidopa/levodopa CR (Sinemet CR), benserazide/levodopa (available in other countries as Madopar or Prolopa), selegiline (Eldepryl), and rasagiline (Azilect), as well as the dopamine agonists (Parlodel, Permax, Mirapex, Requip), can induce vivid dreams, hallucinations, paranoia, and delusions. (An *agonist* is a drug that enhances the actions of another biochemical.) The dopamine agonists "trick" the brain into reacting to them as it would to dopamine, so these drugs cause effects similar to the effects of dopamine. Dopamine agonists, then, make up to some extent for the dopamine shortage in Parkinson's disease. As mentioned above, these drugs cause ICDs much more often than levodopa, are more likely than levodopa to cause hallucinations, and can also cause fatigue, sleepiness, or agitation. (For more information on drugs and the side effects of drugs, see Chapters 11, 12, and 13.)

The drugs tolcapone (Tasmar) and entacapone (Comtan) may also produce behavioral effects, since they increase the amount of levodopa available. The drug amantadine (Symmetrel) can cause confusion; it should be started slowly and carefully monitored, particularly in people who have a history of kidney disease.

Sedatives and Tranquilizers. A number of medications that have sedating effects may also contribute to behavioral changes or psychiatric symptoms when used with Parkinson's medication. These include sleeping pills, drugs to reduce anxiety, and muscle relaxants.

IN THE NEXT CHAPTER we discuss young-onset Parkinson's disease, which is not nearly as common as Parkinson's that develops in later life. Then in Chapter 8 we turn to a discussion of what goes into making a diagnosis of true Parkinson's disease, and in Chapters 9 and 10 we describe some diseases that may be mistaken for Parkinson's disease, or vice versa.

CHAPTER 7

Young-Onset Parkinson's Disease

- *What are the differences between young-onset and later-onset Parkinson's disease?*
- *What special concerns need to be addressed by young adults diagnosed with Parkinson's?*

When a person younger than fifty develops symptoms of Parkinson's disease, he or she faces medical, social, and economic issues quite different from those faced by people whose Parkinson's appears at a later age. In this chapter we discuss some of these issues. (Note that *young-onset Parkinson's disease* is entirely separate from what we sometimes call *early Parkinson's disease,* the symptoms of which are described in Chapter 3. Every person who has Parkinson's experiences early Parkinson's disease following the onset of symptoms.)

WHAT IS YOUNG-ONSET PARKINSON'S DISEASE?

As noted in Chapter 2, the average age of onset of Parkinson's is sixty. In the medical literature, *young-onset Parkinson's* often refers to disease in which symptoms first appear in a person before age forty, but we generally consider age fifty the upper limit for young onset, so in this book we define young-onset Parkinson's disease as disease that causes symptoms in a person older than twenty and younger than fifty.

It is highly unusual for Parkinson's symptoms to develop in someone younger than twenty or thirty, and such symptoms most likely do not represent true Parkinson's disease. The term *juvenile-onset parkinsonism* is usually used for the rare cases of persons diagnosed with Parkinson's before the age of twenty.

We want to emphasize that young-onset Parkinson's disease is not common. About 10 to 15 percent of people who come to our centers for consultations about Parkinson's-like symptoms are found to have young-onset Parkinson's (onset before age fifty), but this proportion is larger than for the population at large because we work in special referral centers for people who have Parkinson's. In the general community, the actual percentage of people who have Parkinson's who develop symptoms before age fifty is about 5 percent.

In the past ten years, exciting new information has begun to accumulate about genetic influences in Parkinson's. As we already discussed in Chapter 2, Parkinson's is not an inherited disorder in most families. While we have learned much about certain genes that are associated with parkinsonism in rare families, we still do not know exactly how these genes work in the brain to cause Parkinson's disease.

What we have learned is that young-onset Parkinson's disease is more likely to be associated with a genetic abnormality. Young-onset Parkinson's (particularly when there is a family history of Parkinson's disease and symptoms began before age forty) is often associated with the so-called recessively inherited genes such as Parkin, DJ-1, and PINK1. ("Recessively inherited" means occurring in siblings but not passed directly from one generation to the next; a child has a one in four chance of inheriting the disease if both parents "carry" the gene but do not have the disease.) The first of these genes to be discovered was Parkin. This gene was initially found in young Japanese patients, but has since been described in people who have Parkinson's from a wide variety of ethnic backgrounds all over the world.

Although doctors can order a genetic test to look for the Parkin gene, this is not currently recommended. A person who has the genetic abnormality typically has two abnormal Parkin genes, and the nature of the abnormality or mutation in each may be the same or different. The importance of having only one abnormal gene (i.e., a "carrier" state) is unknown. One possibility is that this could predispose individuals to later development of more typical Parkinson's disease. Testing for the abnormal Parkin gene is a very complicated task, and it is easy for a laboratory to miss the abnormality. Whether a person who has young-onset Parkinson's does or does not have the Parkin gene doesn't affect treatment. Additional abnormal genes associated with young-onset Parkinson's are certain to be discovered.

Although Parkin, DJ-1, and PINK1 are all relatively recent discoveries, there is a beginning understanding of how these abnormal genes affect the brain's dopaminergic system and cause the symptoms of Parkinson's. It is hoped that as these basic genotypical/biochemical pathways are better understood, more treatments specifically directed at these genetic forms of parkinsonism will be achieved.

It has been astounding to learn that these recessive forms of parkinsonism, with very few differences from typical sporadic Parkinson's (e.g., younger age of onset, perhaps slower progression, perhaps more tremor, perhaps more dystonic postures), can manifest as Parkinson's. The symptoms, progression, and response to dopaminergic treatment is the same. We dwell on these facts because they illustrate the pace and scope of current research in Parkinson's disease and are cause for real hope for future treatments.

SYMPTOMS OF YOUNG-ONSET VERSUS LATER-ONSET PARKINSON'S

Generally, symptoms in people who have young-onset Parkinson's are similar to symptoms in those with later-onset disease, although studies comparing the two groups have identified some differences. For example, people who have young-onset Parkinson's disease seem to be more likely to have a "tremor predominant presentation." In other words, tremor is often a more prominent early symptom in young-onset Parkinson's than in later-onset disease.

Dystonia, or abnormal Parkinson's muscle spasms, may show up earlier in the course of disease in young-onset Parkinson's, too. The dystonia may involve curling of the toes, with the big toe pointing up, or turning in of the ankle. This muscle cramping may cause discomfort and may interfere with such activities as walking. In later-onset Parkinson's disease these symptoms generally do not appear until later in the course of illness, after medication has been started, and then most often at times when the effects of levodopa wear off (e.g., first thing in the morning; see Chapter 4). In some individuals, especially those with young-onset Parkinson's, the dystonia may begin before the use of levodopa is started.

Some studies have also reported that people who have young-onset Parkinson's are more likely to develop drug-induced dyskinesia and motor fluctuations, and these may occur quite soon (within the first year) after levodopa is begun. (More information on these symptoms is given in Chapter 12.) At this time, however, we don't know whether the disease of persons who have young-onset Parkinson's progresses any differently from later-onset disease.

Diagnostic Difficulties

Many people who have young-onset Parkinson's understandably become frustrated when they cannot get an accurate diagnosis, even when they see one doctor after another. Although a person in his or her thirties may have a typical-looking resting tremor and stiffness and slowness of one hand that appear exactly like classic early Parkinson's disease, most physicians are simply not likely to consider Parkinson's as a diagnosis in young adults. When the typical resting tremor is absent, it is even less likely that physicians will consider a Parkinson's diagnosis. The symptoms of early Parkinson's disease may even be mistaken for psychological problems such as depression or anxiety. These misdiagnoses frequently result in years of unnecessary diagnostic investigations and well-intentioned but misguided therapies.

Young adults who have Parkinson's symptoms may benefit from visiting a center for the study of movement disorders. (See Chapter 1 for information on how to locate one of these centers or a neurologist who specializes in diagnosing and treating movement disorders.) Because young-onset Parkinson's disease is not common, a thorough examination by a neurologist with extensive experience in Parkinson's disease is essential for the young patient. Physicians often use blood tests and imaging studies (computerized axial tomography [CAT] scans and magnetic resonance imaging [MRI] of the brain) to identify causes for these symptoms other than Parkinson's.

Coping

Adjusting to a diagnosis of Parkinson's disease is always difficult, but adults in their thirties or forties confront problems that are fundamentally different from those faced by people in their sixties or seventies. Both younger people and older people have to adjust to the idea of chronic illness, but the younger person often has the additional responsibility of a young family and a career.

Once a diagnosis is made, the effects of the disease on a career path can be planned for, because we have information about many of the symptoms of Parkinson's. People need to consider the effects of Parkinson's symptoms on their career and on their plans to start or add to a family. And they need to consider carefully what they will do about obtaining and retaining medical and disability insurance, which becomes increasingly significant when someone has a chronic illness.

Medical insurance purchased through an employer continues even after a diagnosis of chronic illness, as long as employment continues. Even after employment ends, the COBRA laws (in the United States) allow an individual to continue medical coverage for a period of time, as long as she or he pays the monthly premiums. Purchasing new health insurance after a diagnosis of Parkinson's often means paying higher premiums. Disability insurance is also more expensive (sometimes prohibitively expensive) after a diagnosis has been made. This is why many insurance agents recommend that healthy people—even young healthy people—purchase disability insurance before an accident occurs or an illness is diagnosed.

Women

Young women with Parkinson's disease have their own set of issues to deal with. For example, women who are still menstruating often report that their menstrual cycle affects their Parkinson's symptoms.

Some say that just prior to menstruation, their symptoms worsen and their tremor and slowness increase. Others report the opposite, with improvement in their symptoms just before menstruation.

It is helpful if a woman observes the severity of her symptoms during the course of her menstrual cycle; some women find it easiest to make notes on a calendar, charting good days and bad days. A woman and her physician can use this information to plan the medication regimen. If her Parkinson's symptoms predictably worsen at a particular time of the month, she may be able to take additional medication then. Or if the side effects from medications, such as drug-induced dyskinesia, predictably worsen for a few days, perhaps the medications can be lowered in conjunction with this phase of the menstrual cycle.

We have only incomplete information about how estrogen and Parkinson's symptoms are related, so we cannot give any definitive advice for women with Parkinson's who need to make decisions about taking estrogens, such as the use of estrogen replacement therapy following menopause. At this time, women should make this decision weighing the same variables of risk and benefit that women without Parkinson's must consider. There is much interest in studies now being conducted to determine how estrogen affects the severity of tremor, slowness, and gait difficulties and to evaluate whether estrogen might play a role as a protective factor in Parkinson's disease.

Because Parkinson's disease generally begins after the onset of menopause, pregnancy is not usually an issue for women with Parkinson's. Nonetheless, a small number of women with Parkinson's disease have become pregnant and have delivered normal babies.

The decision to proceed with a pregnancy is a complex one, not only emotionally but, for a woman with Parkinson's disease, medically. Some women who become pregnant find their Parkinson's symptoms get worse during the pregnancy and do not fully return to the prepregnancy level of severity after the baby is born. It is impossible to say whether this is an effect of the pregnancy or the natural progression of the illness. In fact, pregnancy during Parkinson's disease is so uncommon that we don't have enough information to state with certainty what effect pregnancy has on the course of the illness.

Any potential effects of antiparkinson medications on the developing fetus must also be considered. There is currently no evidence that taking carbidopa/levodopa during pregnancy has harmful effects on the fetus. We have less information on other Parkinson's medications—and more cause for concern. Therefore, we advise avoiding all other antiparkinson medication during pregnancy.

In summary, the hormonal changes associated with menstruation, pregnancy, menopause, the use of oral contraceptives or hormone replacement therapy, or surgical removal of the ovaries (oophorectomy) may affect the symptoms of women with Parkinson's disease. Further study is needed to characterize these hormonal effects.

Families

One question concerning children, whether biological or adopted, applies equally to the young man and the young woman considering parenthood. What effect will the Parkinson's symptoms have on a young parent and on the family as a whole? People must carefully consider their individual circumstances. If you are in this position, you may want to talk to a physician experienced in treating people who have Parkinson's disease and consider family counseling before committing to starting or enlarging a family.

Parkinson's nearly always affects both the person who has the disease and the spouse. Adult children, too, often become involved in the care of an older parent with Parkinson's disease. In the case of young-onset Parkinson's, though, the disease can have a serious impact on the lives of young children in the family. The emotional needs of the young children of an individual with Parkinson's disease should not be overlooked. Depending upon the circumstances, family counseling could include the children. Furthermore, a strong marital relationship is generally better nurtured when the spouse of a young person who has Parkinson's has a support system, formal or informal.

Career Issues

Like later-onset Parkinson's disease, young-onset Parkinson's progresses relatively slowly. Many people who have Parkinson's continue to work and advance in their careers for many years following the onset of their symptoms. Indeed, continued engagement in a full life, including family, career, and hobbies, is critical to a healthy adjustment to the diagnosis of Parkinson's disease. We discussed work and career issues related to Parkinson's disease in Chapter 1. This discussion applies regardless of when Parkinson's disease begins.

A common source of concern for people who have Parkinson's is the need to tell family members, coworkers, and employers about the disease. There is no one correct approach to this task. People who have Parkinson's need to decide, either by themselves or in consultation with family, friends, and doctors, how to handle information about their illness. However, excessive efforts to hide the diagnosis are often counterproductive (see Chapter 1).

The Americans with Disabilities Act may provide some relief from anxiety about informing coworkers and employers. Under this act, Parkinson's disease is considered a disability. This means that if you work for a company with more than fifteen employees, and if you have informed your employer that you have Parkinson's, your employer is obliged to make "reasonable accommodations" for your disability. You cannot be fired because you have Parkinson's disease.

SERVICES NEEDED BY YOUNGER PEOPLE

Most community and medical resources for those with Parkinson's disease are geared to older people, and younger people may find it difficult to get the assistance they need. Young adults may feel out of place when they attend a Parkinson's support group in which the majority of people who have Parkinson's and their caregivers are in their sixties and seventies, for example. Also, many medical services, including rehabilitation therapy and routine visits to the doctor, pose scheduling difficulties for people who have full-time jobs—difficulties that don't exist for the retired person.

Various national Parkinson's foundations are now organizing young patient support groups. We should also note, though, that many younger people have benefited from being part of support groups composed of people of various ages. Most of the difficulties of dealing with Parkinson's symptoms are shared by everyone with the disease, regardless of age.

TREATMENT CONCERNS

The physician's foremost concern when Parkinson's appears in people in their thirties or forties is how to manage the symptoms to provide the patient with the best possible quality of life for the longest time. After years of use, antiparkinson medications may produce some undesirable side effects (see Chapter 12), some of which are more disruptive for an individual still in the workplace than for someone who is retired.

Many of the serious side effects of antiparkinson medications occur after long use. The simplest way to avoid these side effects is to reduce the amount of time a person is using the medication. There is a balancing act here, however. Younger persons generally have more life ahead of them and therefore more opportunity to develop these long-term problems, and thus delaying the start of medications would be best. On the other hand, a younger person probably still has family and career responsibilities that are harder to fulfill with Parkinson's symptoms in full bloom, and medication would be especially beneficial for them at this time.

If you find yourself in this position, be sure to check with your physician about the variety of drugs available and their effects. Finding the right balance is a continuing process worked out between the patient and the physician.

Anyone's overall health can be improved by paying special attention to nutrition, managing stress, and keeping physically fit, and all the effects of these activities are desirable (see Chapter 14). Sometimes such measures can help handle symptoms so well that the use of medications can be reduced or delayed. And, as noted above, when Parkinson's disease starts at an early age, delaying medications is a great advantage. On the other hand, the management of Parkinson's should concentrate on current quality of life and not over-emphasize possible future problems that may or may not develop. Some younger patients, concerned about the later development of complications of medications or the misguided and incorrect beliefs that dopaminergic therapy is somehow toxic or loses effect after the first five years of use, delay treatment with the result that they experience unnecessary disability. The consequences of delaying treatment too long can be just as or more disruptive than the early development of drug-related side effects. A balanced approach to initiating treatment is necessary; not necessarily starting at the very earliest stages when the symptoms cause no impact whatsoever on function or quality of life, and not delaying beyond a time when the symptoms are having this impact.

The younger person who has Parkinson's disease should try to maintain a wellspring of hope, fed by the realization that he or she will be the beneficiary of the rapid progress now being made in both the understanding and the management of Parkinson's disease.

Part III

Diagnosing Parkinson's Disease

CHAPTER 8

How a Diagnosis Is Made

- *How is a diagnosis of Parkinson's disease made?*
- *What symptoms suggest a diagnosis other than true Parkinson's?*

Parkinson's disease is just one of several neurologic movement disorders that produce similar symptoms. The "cousins" of Parkinson's disease are referred to variously as *Parkinson's-plus, atypical Parkinson's,* and other causes of *parkinsonism*; typically when we first see patients, if the diagnosis is uncertain we will inform them that they have parkinsonism, with the additional explanation that Parkinson's disease is the commonest cause of this presentation but that other diseases can also result in the same presentation. In some of these diseases people quickly become totally disabled; in others, the disease progresses extremely slowly; and in yet others, illness is chronic (always present) and may have more severe symptoms as time goes on. Because the natural history, or progression, of these diseases varies greatly, proper diagnosis is crucial. People need to know which disease they have.

THE MEDICAL EXAMINATION

When someone goes to see a doctor with concerns about specific symptoms he or she is experiencing, the doctor asks questions about the person's medical history and then performs a physical examination.

After listening to and examining the patient, the doctor decides what the diagnostic possibilities are (this is called making a *differential diagnosis*) and then, if necessary or helpful, the doctor orders tests designed to confirm or highly support a diagnosis. Diagnostic tests include blood tests, x-rays, and computerized axial tomography (CAT) and magnetic resonance imaging (MRI) scans. Once the diagnosis has been established, the doctor can determine which therapy is best to treat the patient's illness and its symptoms.

The Neurologic Examination

When performing a neurologic examination to evaluate a patient with a movement disorder, the doctor takes a history and performs a physical examination. The doctor asks the patient and the family members or friends about symptoms (see below) and observes the patient, asking him or her to walk around the room, sit down, stand up, turn around, and so on. The neurologic exam is a thorough evaluation of the nervous system. In particular, the neurologist observes aspects of the patient's movement, coordination, and balance:

—Is there slowness of movement when the patient moves his hands and fingers or taps his toes?
—Does the patient swing her arms fully and equally while walking?
—Does the patient have particular difficulty turning, and is there any alteration in the size of his stride?
—Does the patient freeze in place or "get stuck" to the floor?
—Does the patient have any characteristic alterations of facial expression and speech quality?

Diagnostic Tests

Unfortunately, there is no diagnostic test that can confirm Parkinson's disease. This remains a true statement despite the increasingly widespread use of dopamine imaging technology (DATScan), which will be discussed later. Laboratory testing of the blood of patients with the symptoms typical of Parkinson's only rarely uncovers any abnormality. Electroencephalograms (EEGs) record some aspects of brain electrical activity, but they are not effective in spotting Parkinson's.

On the other hand, some tests can be used to *rule out* Parkinson's, such as genetic or blood tests that indicate the person has Huntington's disease or Wilson's disease. Neurologists do not routinely order these types of additional diagnostic tests, but they use the tests selectively when they observe atypical symptoms. Neuropsychological testing of patients with cognitive dysfunction or behavioral alteration may help identify particular patterns of other diseases, such as Alzheimer's, and may narrow down the possible diagnoses, but people who have early Parkinson's usually show only minor abnormalities on these tests (see Chapter 6).

The MRI and CAT scans of the brain produce remarkable and exquisite anatomic pictures, and the radiologist can find areas with anomalies that might indicate brain tumors, strokes (cerebral infarction), or abnormal enlargement of the fluid-filled spaces in the brain (hydrocephalus). Imaging scans can be useful in helping the physician rule out other causes for the symptoms. But the MRI and CAT scans of the brain of people who have Parkinson's disease appear normal. The brain changes that create neurodegenerative diseases such as Parkinson's are microscopic, on a chemical level, and are generally not revealed by these scans, but newer methods of evaluating MRI scans may provide ways of distinguishing some atypical parkinsonisms from Parkinson's disease and may eventually even be able to distinguish people who have Parkinson's disease from people who do not have Parkinson's disease.

Certain types of positron emission tomography (PET) scan and single photon emission computed tomography (SPECT) scan are used to assess the dopamine system in the brain. PET scans are not widely available and are mainly used in research. The types of SPECT Scan that assess the transporter for dopamine in the brain are being introduced in North America, and have been available for some time in Europe. Importantly, the findings from these imaging techniques are generally similar for Parkinson's disease and for most other causes of parkinsonism, so they are not a way of narrowing the diagnosis any further than can a neurologist experienced in assessing these disorders. In fact, the SPECT Scan cannot distinguish the various "cousins" of

Parkinson's (atypical parkinsonism, parkinsonism plus) and therefore it is not useful for eliminating these more serious forms of parkinsonism. In the United States, the DATScan (SPECT) is being promoted as a diagnostic tool that can distinguish essential tremor (ET) from parkinsonism—a differential diagnosis we will discuss later. Another test that is used widely in some countries in Europe in the investigation of Parkinson's is transcranial ultrasound (using the same technology as radar or sonar). Most people who have Parkinson's have an increased echo signal in the area of the brain that contains the dopamine cells (substantia nigra), while it is claimed that many of the other causes of parkinsonism are not associated with this change. It should be pointed out that 10 percent of the normal population are found to have the same increased echo signal. The utility of this tool in the evaluation of patients and even for research and screening large populations remains uncertain.

The results of diagnostic tests, then, are more likely either to point to a diagnosis other than Parkinson's disease or to be inconclusive— they do not show any abnormal results that can be identified as due to a specific disease process.

PARKINSON'S DISEASE: A CLINICAL DIAGNOSIS

With no diagnostic tests to provide specific answers, physicians must base their diagnosis of Parkinson's on judgment. Physicians are intimately familiar with the characteristic history and the signs and symptoms found when examining a person who has Parkinson's. They then must judge how closely the history of symptoms and the neurologic findings (from the physical examination) of any specific person match those of typical Parkinson's disease. This determination through the judgment of the doctor (the clinician) is called a *clinical diagnosis*.

Accurate diagnosis of neurologic movement disorders is tricky, even in the best of hands. As many as one in five persons with Parkinson's receives a misdiagnosis. (How do we know that one person in five is likely to be misdiagnosed? This information comes from studies involving long-term follow-up of patients and confirmation of the diagnosis by autopsy.) Parkinson's disease and the diseases that masquerade as Parkinson's pose a challenge even for the experienced physician, and if a doctor has not had experience with these other diseases and with Parkinson's, diagnosis can be very challenging indeed.

The chance of arriving at the correct diagnosis is considerably improved when the patient consults a physician experienced in neurology and specifically in the neurologic field of movement disorders. People who have parkinsonian symptoms should expect their doctor to listen carefully to their and their families' description of symptoms and to conduct a thorough neurologic examination. Such an examination includes observing the patient's finger, hand, and foot movements and observing the patient walk, turn, and resist postural challenges (pushing or pulling the patient to see if he or she can avoid falling). The doctor also observes the patient to see whether any abnormal movements (e.g., tremor) are visible and whether the patient can easily arise from a chair. Facial expression, eye movements, and speech are examined. The doctor flexes and extends (bends) the patient's neck, arms, wrists, and legs to examine for abnormal muscle tone. Strength and coordination of the arms are evaluated. The cognitive (mental) function of the patient is also assessed. Figures 8.1 through 8.9 illustrate these examination procedures.

When people have symptoms of slowness, rigidity, and characteristic alterations of their gait, they undoubtedly have *parkinsonism*. The question is whether or not they have true Parkinson's disease. As mentioned above, the disorders that resemble Parkinson's share many of the same symptoms and signs: tremor, rigidity, slowness (bradykinesia), problems with posture and walking, and balance problems.

Sometimes all the doctor can do is wait for several months then reexamine the patient to determine whether the changes in the symptoms are typical of true Parkinson's. Delay in diagnosis can be frustrating for both patients and physicians. But Parkinson's is a serious disease, and the diagnosis must be accurate so the doctor can choose appropriate therapies and people can have an idea of how their disease will change in the future.

We have found the observations made by the person with symptoms and by her or his friends and family particularly important, often

FIGURES 8.1 AND 8.2 The neurologist is testing to see whether the patient has balance problems. In this test the physician stands directly behind the patient and pulls him backward, to find out whether the patient can maintain his balance. In this case the patient's balance is impaired and he falls backward.

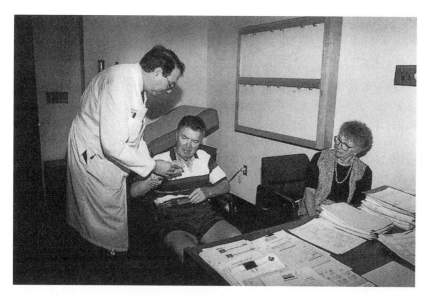

FIGURE 8.3 The neurologist moves the patient's wrist to test for range of motion and determine whether cogwheel rigidity is present.

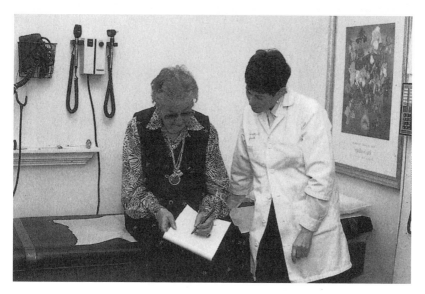

FIGURE 8.4 The patient is providing a handwriting sample so the neurologist can determine whether micrographia (small handwriting) is present.

FIGURE 8.5 The patient is receiving counseling about drug therapy from the neurologist.

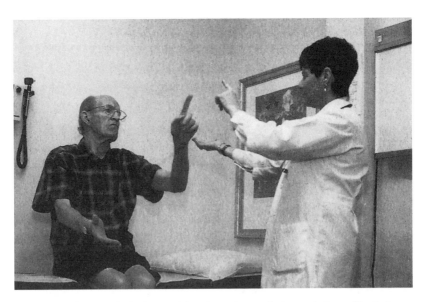

FIGURE 8.6 The neurologist is examining the patient to find out whether a kinetic tremor (see page 137) is present. In this maneuver the patient touches the neurologist's finger and then touches his nose and then the neurologist's finger again.

FIGURE 8.7 The neurologist is examining the patient to see whether her ability to open and close her hand is normal, or whether there is evidence of slowness (bradykinesia). This patient exhibits a "masked" face, which means that the person's face has a tendency to be without expression. In other words, she does not have normal spontaneous movement of her facial muscles, so her face does not reflect her emotions very well. A masked face can be mistaken for disinterest, apathy, dementia, depression, or even hostility. The masked face reflects none of these emotional states but instead reflects the effect of Parkinson's disease on the facial muscles of some patients.

containing the seeds of the correct diagnosis. As we noted in earlier chapters, friends or family members may notice the initial Parkinson's tremor even before the affected person does. They may spot the characteristic Parkinson's posture and gait. Family members may also identify symptoms indicating that Parkinson's is not the right diagnosis. They make observations such as, "I just don't think my brother has Parkinson's disease, because I have been to support groups with him, and the other people there look very different from him."

In the rest of this chapter we look at some of the questions and answers that might lead toward or away from a diagnosis of Parkinson's disease.

FIGURE 8.8 The neurologist is examining the patient to find out whether she is able to rise from a chair with her arms crossed. Many patients with axial bradykinesia and rigidity have difficulty rising from a chair without pushing up with their hands.

FIGURE 8.9 The neurologist is examining the patient to find out whether she has normal finger dexterity (movement).

Questions Leading to a Diagnosis of Parkinson's Disease

Here and in the next section, we provide lists of the common questions a doctor asks when a patient complains of symptoms of a neurologic movement disorder. A *yes* answer to the questions in this first list of questions, addressed to the patient, may suggest a diagnosis of Parkinson's disease.

—Have you experienced the onset of a one-sided (unilateral) tremor (typically with the limb at rest or in the arm while walking) within the last year or two that has become progressively worse?
—Do you notice awkwardness when using your hands to fasten buttons, brush your teeth, comb your hair, beat eggs, or manipulate a knife and fork?
—Does one of your legs drag or move slowly when you are walking?
—Have you noticed that you seem to stoop when you stand or walk?
—Does one of your arms fail to swing when you walk?
—Has your voice changed, lost its force, or become softer?
—Have family members noticed that your facial expression has changed?
—Have they noticed that you do not seem to smile as much as before?
—Have your eyes and face developed a staring quality?

If a patient answers yes to any of these questions, the doctor will ask whether the severity of these symptoms has remained the same, worsened, or improved with time, because Parkinson's symptoms gradually progress. (Symptoms of early, moderate, and advanced Parkinson's are detailed in Chapters 3, 4, and 5.)

Questions Leading Away from a Diagnosis of Parkinson's Disease

As noted above, and indeed throughout this book, Parkinson's is one of a group of diseases that share symptoms. The "cousins" of Parkinson's disease include progressive supranuclear palsy (PSP), multiple system atrophy (MSA), dementia with Lewy bodies, corticobasal degeneration (CBD), multiple small strokes, and Alzheimer's disease. (See Chapters 9 and 10 for more information about these diseases.) A yes answer to any of the following questions may lead toward a diagnosis of one of these other diseases and away from a diagnosis of Parkinson's disease.

—Did your symptoms begin abruptly after a surgical procedure?

—Do you have a history of multiple strokes?

—Is there a history of an illness like this in your parents, grandparents, children, or siblings (we now recognize several genetic forms of Parkinson's disease, as well, so a family history may not be as helpful as it was once thought to be in distinguishing Parkinson's from other forms of parkinsonism; in fact, a family history is more common in Parkinson's than in the various causes of parkinsonism listed above)?

—Have you been exposed to toxins (for example in the workplace), including manganese? Suffered from carbon monoxide intoxication? Used illicit drugs? Or taken any major tranquilizers such as chlorpromazine (Thorazine), thioridazine (Mellaril), haloperidol (Haldol), perphenazine/amitriptyline (Triavil), or trifluoperazine (Stelazine)?

—Have you taken any of the "atypical" tranquilizers such as risperidone (Risperdal), olanzapine (Zyprexa), quetiapine (Seroquel), aripiprazole (Abilify), or ziprasidone (Geodon)?

—Have you taken the gastrointestinal medication metoclopramide (Reglan)?

—Have your family or friends mentioned that your personality seems to have changed?

—Do you find you can't remember things that just happened?

—Has your family indicated that you seem more confused than usual?

—Do you have trouble moving your eyes, or do you have any general visual disturbance?

—Soon after these symptoms started, did you often have trouble with your balance or have problems with falling?

—Soon after these symptoms started, did you develop difficulty with your speech?

—Soon after these symptoms started, did you develop difficulty with swallowing?

—Before or soon after these symptoms started, did you experience faintness on standing up, problems controlling urination, or sexual impotence (males)?

—Do you have mostly slow movements, stiffness, loss of facial expression, difficulty with walking, but no tremor whatsoever?

If the person does not have a characteristic resting tremor, Parkinson's disease is less likely. If the symptoms are completely symmetrical from the onset, rather than being more prominent on one side of the body, Parkinson's disease may be less likely (although some people who have Parkinson's do have symmetrical symptoms and some with atypical parkinsonism may be very asymmetrical). Also, if symptoms do not respond to antiparkinson medications, the problem probably is not Parkinson's disease. Certain drugs, particularly those used in treating schizophrenia, also can cause parkinsonism, but they do not cause Parkinson's disease.

Over time, the person who has mild parkinsonism usually develops additional symptoms that contain vital clues to accurate diagnosis. The following summary provides information about some symptoms and the Parkinson's-plus disorders they may indicate. (See Chapters 9 and 10 for more information on all these disorders.)

1. Problems with cognitive function, including memory, personality changes, and falling, don't usually occur until people have had Parkinson's for many years, perhaps decades. Some families notice that the person with symptoms is becoming forgetful, particularly of recent events. For example, she or he may be able to recall events of forty to fifty years ago with great accuracy, but confuses recent events. Personality changes may show up in various ways, such as increased passivity or increased aggressiveness or less interest in hobbies and socialization. All these emerging symptoms may indicate such disorders as dementia with Lewy bodies or Alzheimer's disease.

2. The person with symptoms and the family members may notice that he or she seems to have difficulty looking down at the food on a plate or difficulty seeing the steps when attempting to walk

up or down a flight of stairs. These eye movement abnormalities coupled with mild parkinsonism and a very early onset of spontaneous falling suggest progressive supranuclear palsy (see Chapter 10).

3. Some people have early signs of dysfunction of the autonomic nervous system. These include serious urinary problems, feeling faint on standing up (because of a sudden drop in blood pressure), and, in men, difficulty achieving an erection. These symptoms may be an indication of multiple system atrophy (see Chapter 10).

The following questions help the doctor distinguish atypical Parkinson's from true Parkinson's disease.

—difficulty moving his or her eyes up and down?
—prominent slurring of the speech early in the course of illness?
—a prominent tremor when reaching for objects, but not when the hands are at rest?
—severe gait impairment with a frequent tendency to lose balance and fall?
—faintness or dizziness when rising from a chair? If so, is the faintness accompanied by alterations of blood pressure?
—any unusual involuntary movements (in the absence of antiparkinson drug use), such as jerking, writhing, dance-like, or twisting movements or chewing movements of the mouth?

Again, a *yes* answer to any of these questions suggests the person has a disease or illness other than Parkinson's disease.

IN THIS CHAPTER we have begun the process of describing how a physician makes a diagnosis of Parkinson's. Because distinguishing between Parkinson's disease and other types of parkinsonism in other neurologic disorders is so important, and sometimes so difficult, in the next two chapters we take a closer look at these other illnesses sometimes mistaken for Parkinson's disease, and vice versa.

CHAPTER 9

Types of Parkinsonism

- *How can the physician distinguish between Parkinson's disease and other causes of parkinsonism?*
- *What is MPTP-induced parkinsonism, and why is it important?*
- *How do strokes cause parkinsonism?*
- *Can head injury cause Parkinson's disease?*
- *Which drugs can cause parkinsonian symptoms?*

Parkinsonism, as we have noted in earlier chapters, is a general term for the TRAP symptoms of Parkinson's disease: tremor, rigidity, akinesia (or bradykinesia), and postural instability. Not every person with these symptoms has Parkinson's disease, however. Any neurologic disorder that affects the dopamine system or its downstream connections will cause similar symptoms. Because a diagnosis of Parkinson's disease is a *clinical* diagnosis (as we saw in Chapter 8), based primarily on a person's symptoms and medical history rather than on the results of a diagnostic test, and because so many disorders cause these same symptoms, diagnosis of a disease that is causing parkinsonism can be difficult.

Patients and family members often help physicians arrive at an accurate diagnosis of Parkinson's disease by describing which symptoms the patient does and does not have, as well as when and how the symptoms began and whether they have become worse. In this chapter and the next we give a detailed description of disorders that are similar to and often confused with Parkinson's disease. Our aim is to make patients and families aware that diagnosis is difficult in part because of the many possible causes of these symptoms. In no way are we suggesting that patients should engage in self-diagnosis or that family members should decide what the patient's problem is. A careful medical history and neurologic examination, combined with the passage of enough time to indicate how the symptoms are progressing, generally lead to an accurate medical diagnosis. When there is any doubt about the diagnosis, a physician experienced in neurology, and specifically in the field of movement disorders, can often help (see Chapter 1).

PARKINSONISM CAUSED BY MPTP
(METHYL PHENYL TETRAHYDROPYRIDINE)

One form of parkinsonism that has generated a great deal of scientific and public interest is MPTP-induced parkinsonism. In his book *The Frozen Addicts,* William Langston presents the case of a young man in his twenties who became ill and, over a short time, developed a severe case of parkinsonism and became immobilized. The young man ultimately died. The reason for his illness was unclear, although illegal drugs were suspected.

Sometime later, in northern California, a group of adults in their twenties, thirties, and forties who were using illegal drugs developed the same illness. Their symptoms became severe within weeks to months, rather than the years and decades typical of Parkinson's disease. They became relatively frozen and immobile, their speech became severely impaired, they developed difficulty walking, and they were unable to care for themselves because they moved so slowly. The neurologist who examined them observed that their parkinsonian symptoms were striking—and odd. For instance, the symptoms occurred in relatively young people and rapidly developed into serious disability. After a great deal of medical sleuthing, scientists found that MPTP (methyl phenyl tetrahydropyridine) was the culprit. While attempting to manufacture a mind-altering drug, an illegal drug producer had accidentally made bad batches containing MPTP, which a number of people had injected.

The importance of the MPTP story goes far beyond the "frozen addicts." Other drugs produce symptoms of Parkinson's because they block dopamine receptors or deplete brain dopamine, preventing dopamine from transmitting nerve signals from the brain to the muscles. Whereas these drugs don't actually change brain structure, MPTP does: it injures the dopamine-producing cells in the part of the brain that is affected in Parkinson's disease. Although its importance for Parkinson's disease was discovered through tragic circumstances, MPTP provides us with a research model of Parkinson's disease. MPTP is used to study mechanisms of nerve cell death that may occur in Parkinson's and to test new drugs in the laboratory.

The MPTP story remains an important historical event. However, it also illustrates how science and research explore an idea and move on. We learned an enormous amount of information about how MPTP induces acute dopaminergic cell damage and the symptoms of parkinsonism, but we also learned that MPTP-induced parkinsonism is not Parkinson's. Although this has provided an excellent animal model to study treatments for symptoms of Parkinson's, we have been increasingly frustrated by the failure of predictions from the MPTP model to be successful in patients when it comes to developing treatments that slow the progression of the disease. Many drugs have successfully modified MPTP-induced parkinsonism in animals but have failed in people who have early Parkinson's. This has led to the search for new animal models of Parkinson's to develop more successful drugs.

As noted in Chapter 2, the MPTP story has also influenced our ideas about the cause of Parkinson's, suggesting that unknown environmental toxins that we eat or breathe could damage dopamine-producing cells and thus cause Parkinson's disease. Unfortunately, even after years of studies attempting to find a specific environmental toxin, not one has been discovered. The pesticide rotenone has chemical effects similar to those of MPTP and has also been used to create an animal model of Parkinson's, but not all researchers agree on its usefulness. Encouraged by knowledge about the function of the Parkin gene (see Chapter 7), researchers have created an animal model of Parkinson's that uses inhibitors of the ubiquitin-proteasome, which is used by cells to clear or remove damaged or abnormal proteins from the cell. Here too, many other investigators have been unable to reproduce the original findings. If this could be confirmed and reproduced in other animals it is an important discovery, because we know there are naturally occurring proteasome inhibitors in the environment. Parkinson's is generally believed to be a blend of genetic and environmental factors. Some people may have several genes that provide a genetic predisposition to Parkinson's, and the disease might appear if and when they are exposed to the variety of environmental toxins that correlate with those genes.

STROKE

A common cause of parkinsonism but not true Parkinson's disease is cerebrovascular disease, or stroke. There are two types of situations in which people develop parkinsonism related to cerebrovascular disease.

In the first situation, someone suddenly develops signs of a stroke, and parkinsonian symptoms of slowness and rigidity develop along with other neurologic symptoms. The term *stroke* refers to the sudden onset of neurologic symptoms such as weakness, difficulty speaking, or difficulty seeing. The weakness comes on suddenly and usually involves one side of the body, for example the right arm and the right leg. Many people fail to recover fully from a stroke, and they may have residual weakness or clumsiness of a hand or persistent slurred speech. In some people the residual deficit of the stroke may include the slowing of movement, difficulty walking, and rigidity of parkinsonism. People who have a stroke do not usually develop a typical parkinsonian tremor but other kinds of tremor are possible.

A stroke is caused by injury to a region of the brain resulting from inadequate blood flow, either because the blood vessels are blocked or because a blood vessel has broken, with subsequent bleeding into the brain. People who experience a stroke need a thorough neurologic evaluation to determine the cause of the stroke. This is particularly important because in recent years there have been a number of important therapeutic advances to prevent the recurrence of stroke.

The second setting in which cerebrovascular disease contributes to the development of parkinsonism is more common but far more subtle and more difficult to recognize. People go to their doctor because they have a condition that looks like slowly evolving Parkinson's disease, including a gradually progressive shuffling gait with intermittent freezing, loss of balance, rigidity, and slowness of movement. The physician may believe the patient is developing Parkinson's disease, but then finds that the medications used to treat Parkinson's do not relieve the symptoms.

In this situation, MRI scans of the brain can be very helpful. The MRI can demonstrate the presence of multiple tiny strokes that have occurred "silently," without the patient's knowledge. When numerous tiny strokes accumulate in deep brain structures such as the basal ganglia or the white matter, parkinsonism may result. The *basal ganglia* are a group of brain regions closely related to the substantia nigra. Similarly, the *white matter* of the brain contains numerous interconnections between the various motor areas, and disruption of these interconnections may cause parkinsonism (see Chapter 11). If the strokes affect other areas of the brain, they may cause dementia.

This condition is sometimes called *vascular parkinsonism* or, because its signs and symptoms are mostly limited to the legs, *lower-half parkinsonism*. After vascular parkinsonism is diagnosed, people are often surprised to learn that small, silent strokes that have caused no sudden symptoms are producing their neurologic symptoms of parkinsonism or dementia.

People who have multiple strokes of the brain that produce parkinsonism have a difficult problem, since antiparkinson medications generally do not relieve their symptoms. The physician's main role is to take every measure possible to help prevent further strokes. A number of preventive therapies are available after the cause of stroke has been determined. For people who have this disorder, it is always useful to stop smoking, to eat nutritiously, and to keep body weight at an appropriate level. Medications to regulate blood pressure, to change blood coagulability, to lower cholesterol, or to control blood sugar are also helpful in treating cerebrovascular disease.

NORMAL PRESSURE HYDROCEPHALUS

Normal pressure hydrocephalus (NPH) is another uncommon cause of parkinsonism, most often resulting in an abnormal gait similar to the lower-half parkinsonism of multiple strokes. Other symptoms of NPH include urinary difficulties and cognitive or thinking problems. The diagnosis is suggested by a CAT scan or MRI that reveals markedly enlarged ventricles in the brain. This can sometimes be a difficult diagnosis to make or confirm. When correctly diagnosed, patients may benefit from a neurosurgical procedure called a shunt. There has recently been a considerable amount of attention to NPH in the media. But keep in mind that NPH is uncommon, and an experienced physician can distinguish Parkinson's disease from NPH. Gradually progressive resting tremor, bradykinesia, and rigidity on one side of the body are characteristic of Parkinson's disease, but the early symptoms of NPH include a halting gait and urinary urgency and incontinence. The symptoms of NPH are unlikely to respond to antiparkinson medications, and the characteristic finding of enlarged ventricles in the brain, revealed by brain imaging, is not seen in people who have Parkinson's disease.

NPH is very rare, but in those people who truly have this disorder, it can be reversible. Unfortunately, its potential reversibility often leads to overenthusiasm in terms of diagnosis. In addition to the MRI of the brain being useful, a procedure called a "high-volume" spinal tap (lumbar puncture [LP]) may be useful. In this procedure, a large volume of fluid is removed at the time of the lumbar puncture and then the patient is observed one or two hours later to see if any neurologic signs (thinking, memory, gait) improve. This is not a foolproof diagnostic test, but if the neurologist and family agree there is a very positive change and the clinical picture and imaging is compatible with the diagnosis, a neurosurgery consultation to consider a shunt can be useful. A shunt is a procedure in which a tube is inserted into the brain's fluid spaces to drain excess fluid.

If the patient and family do not wish to consider a shunt placement, there is no point in doing the high-volume spinal tap. This diagnostic procedure is done only to screen for the possibility that a shunt might be useful. An alternative approach to a single high-volume spinal tap is a two- or three-day spinal fluid drainage procedure. This approach has been touted as providing a better assessment of whether the placement of a shunt would be helpful. This prolonged spinal drainage requires a one- or two-day stay in the hospital and is associated with a small chance of serious central nervous infection. There is no definite evidence that the procedure is any better than a single high-volume spinal tap. Shunt placement is a surgical procedure with complications possible.

HEAD INJURY

Head injury can cause Parkinson's-like symptoms, but it does not cause Parkinson's disease. The areas of the brain linked to parkinsonism—the basal ganglia and substantia nigra—are located deep in the center of the brain. Head trauma would have to be quite severe to disrupt the dopamine system or its connections in these areas. Minor head trauma is not capable of causing such changes.

Furthermore, the basal ganglia and substantia nigra are surrounded by many other vital neurologic structures, such as the control centers for eye movement and voluntary motor movement and structures related to consciousness. People who develop parkinsonism due to head trauma usually have other symptoms as well: subsequent loss of consciousness, coma, weakness on one side of the body (hemiparesis), disrupted eye movements, and other signs of severe neurologic damage.

In addition, parkinsonism resulting from head trauma is not progressive. In other words, if people survive severe head trauma, their parkinsonian symptoms are most severe immediately after they recover consciousness, then they stabilize or improve. This form of parkinsonism also responds poorly to antiparkinson medication.

Another kind of head trauma associated with parkinsonism is called *dementia pugilistica*. This term describes a condition found in boxers who, after repeated fights and untold numbers of blows to the head, become "punch drunk" and lose cognitive skills, such as memory. Some boxers also develop parkinsonism, with slowness of movement, stiffness, and even tremor as a result of the repeated blows to the head. The cause of these neurologic symptoms is thought to be repeated head trauma with multiple small hemorrhages in the brain in various structures that control movement and thinking. There is increasing interest in the role of repeated concussive head injuries in other sports (e.g., football, hockey) causing similar brain disease, typically associated with cognitive decline. To date there is no evidence that this is a cause of Parkinson's disease, although once again these individuals may have some features of parkinsonism on examination.

Many studies have evaluated the association between head trauma and true Parkinson's disease. Studies of veterans of World War I and

World War II who had received head injuries and who later developed neurologic symptoms provide evidence that head trauma does not cause Parkinson's disease. People who have Parkinson's lose their balance, and the falls that result can cause head injury with or without loss of consciousness. This type of head injury does not increase the rate of progression of the disease.

DRUGS

Parkinsonism can be caused by certain drugs. We have already discussed MPTP-induced parkinsonism. Here we discuss the prescription medications that can induce parkinsonism (Table 9.1). Physicians need to be aware of the potential for drug-induced parkinsonism, since this is usually reversible when the offending medication is discontinued.

Drug-induced parkinsonism may have all the features of true Parkinson's disease, including resting tremor, slowness of movement, decrease in finger and hand dexterity, soft monotonous voice, gait difficulties, balance problems, and cogwheel rigidity.

The most common medications that may cause parkinsonism are the *neuroleptics*, major tranquilizers used to treat such diseases as schizophrenia and psychosis. Neuroleptics block dopamine receptors in the brain and therefore obstruct the function of dopamine. The neuroleptics include chlorpromazine (Thorazine), haloperidol (Haldol), trifluoperazine (Stelazine), perphenazine/amitriptyline (Triavil), and thioridazine (Mellaril).

New medications called *atypical neuroleptics* also block dopamine receptors but are less likely to induce or worsen parkinsonism. The atypical neuroleptics include olanzapine (Zyprexa), risperidone (Risperdal), ziprasidone (Geodon), aripiprazole (Abilify), quetiapine (Seroquel), and clozapine (Clozaril). Although they are less likely to cause parkinsonism than the older typical neuroleptics most of these are still capable of causing this problem. Because of this risk most should not be used in Parkinson's disease with the exception of quetiapine and clozapine.

Minor tranquilizers, such as diazepam (Valium), chlordiazepoxide (Librium), lorazepam (Ativan), alprazolam (Xanax), and temazepam (Restoril), do not cause parkinsonism.

TABLE 9.1
Drugs That May Cause Parkinsonism

Generic name	Trademark name

Major tranquilizers (antipsychotics, neuroleptics)

Acetophenazine maleate	Tindal
Butaperazine maleate	Repoise maleate
Carphenazine maleate	Proketazine
Chlorpromazine	Thorazine
Chlorprothizene	Taractan
Fluphenazine decanoate	Prolixin Decanoate
Fluphenazine enanthate	Prolixin Enanthate
Fluphenazine hydrochloride	Permitil
Fluphenazine hydrochloride	Prolixin
Haloperidol	Haldol
Loxapine	Loxitane
Mesoridazine	Serentil
Molindone hydrochloride	Moban
Perphenazine	Trilafon
Perphenazine/amitryptiline	Triavil
Pimozide	Orap
Piperacetazine*	
Promazine	Sparine
Sulpiride*	
Thioridazine	Mellaril
Thiothixene	Navane
Trifluoperazine	Stelazine

Atypical neuroleptics (newer forms of major tranquilizers)

Aripiprazole	Abilify
Clozapine	Clozaril
Olanzapine	Zyprexa
Quetiapine	Seroquel
Risperidone	Risperdal
Ziprasidone	Geodon

Gastrointestinal motility agent

Metoclopramide	Reglan

Antihypertensives (lower blood pressure)

Reserpine[†]	

(continued)

TABLE 9.1 (CONTINUED)

Generic name	Trademark name
Antiemetics (prevents nausea and vomiting)	
Prochlorperazine	Compazine
Trimethobenzamide	Tigan
Specific calcium channel blockers (used for a variety of indications)	
Flunarizine*	
Cinnarizine*	

*Not marketed in the United States.
†Rare ingredient in various drugs for high blood pressure treatment.

Two drugs used to treat nausea, prochlorperazine (Compazine) and trimethobenzamide (Tigan), and a drug used for gastrointestinal disorders, metoclopramide (Reglan), can also induce parkinsonism. Although not commonly used, an old antihypertensive medication (to lower blood pressure) called reserpine can also induce parkinsonism. Reserpine depletes brain dopamine rather than blocking dopamine receptors. Reserpine is still sometimes found in combination antihypertensives. People taking an antihypertensive who begin developing parkinsonism should find out whether their medication contains reserpine. Tetrabenazine is another drug that works mainly by depleting brain dopamine; this is used in the treatment of movement disorders and the physicians who prescribe this drug should regularly monitor for features of drug-induced parkinsonism.

Although drug-induced parkinsonism can look very similar to Parkinson's disease, some important features can help the physician determine whether the problem might be drug-induced parkinsonism rather than Parkinson's disease. "Red flags" include a history of exposure to potentially offending medications. In drug-related parkinsonism, significant symptoms often develop over a relatively short time, such as two, three, or four months, instead of over a period of years. If the parkinsonian symptoms equally involve both sides of the body at the same time, this is also cause for believing the problem is something other than Parkinson's disease, since Parkinson's symptoms usually develop on one side first.

After drug-induced parkinsonism is diagnosed, many people completely recover when the offending drug is discontinued, although this may take six to twelve months. But some people do not fully recover. Instead, after a period of improvement, their parkinsonian symptoms may again begin to get worse. At first this seems paradoxical, but it has a rather simple explanation. All the drugs with the capacity to cause parkinsonism do so by reducing dopamine transmission between cells within the brain. When a person is at risk of developing Parkinson's disease later in life, exposure to a drug that interferes with the dopamine system may provoke the development of Parkinson's symptoms before the person, without the drug, would have developed symptoms. After a period of improvement, the worsening of the parkinsonism over time may be the course of true Parkinson's disease emerging.

When people who have been diagnosed with Parkinson's disease receive medications listed in Table 9.1, there is a significant risk that their Parkinson's symptoms will rapidly worsen. If possible, these types of drugs should be avoided in all people who have Parkinson's. Nonetheless, there are situations when the use of major tranquilizers is necessary—for example, when hallucinations or delusions become a problem, usually following many years of taking medications for Parkinson's. This is a complex problem that is best managed by physicians with special expertise in Parkinson's disease. The use of the atypical neuroleptics is much preferable to the older major tranquilizers. The patient will need close monitoring for side effects of increasing parkinsonism when taking these types of drugs.

DISCRIMINATING AMONG parkinsonism related to stroke, drug-induced parkinsonism, and Parkinson's disease is often extremely challenging and requires the clinical expertise of a physician who understands the nuances of parkinsonism. In the next chapter the further extent of the challenge emerges, as we consider the full range of atypical parkinsonian syndromes.

CHAPTER 10

Diagnosing Other
Neurologic Problems

- *How can the doctor tell whether I have Parkinson's or one of these other diseases?*

  —*Essential tremor*   —*Wilson's disease*
  —*Huntington's disease*   —*Multiple system atrophy*
  —*Tics*   —*Progressive supranuclear palsy*
  —*Dystonia*   —*Alzheimer's disease*

        In this chapter we discuss neurologic problems often confused with Parkinson's disease, sometimes by patients and sometimes by physicians. Most of these disorders have a whole set of characteristic symptoms.

    As we have noted, the observations of the patient, friends, and family members contain considerable wisdom that can help physicians make an accurate diagnosis. Recently, a young woman brought her grandmother to us, explaining, "I have been to several doctors who insist that she has Parkinson's disease, but I have been reading about Parkinson's disease on the Internet. I don't think my grandmother has it. I think she fits the description of progressive supranuclear palsy. She has difficulty walking, she moves slowly, and she has a lot of trouble moving her eyes." When we examined the grandmother, we were impressed to find that the young woman had correctly diagnosed progressive supranuclear palsy. We relate this story to illustrate the valuable information that patients and family can contribute. Self-diagnosis is to be avoided.

TABLE 10.1
CLUES THAT YOU DON'T HAVE TYPICAL PARKINSON'S DISEASE

Lack of tremor, especially the typical resting tremor
Lack of response to antiparkinson medications
Difficulty with eye movements
Early onset (within two years) of balance problems and falls
Early onset of personality changes
Early onset of forgetfulness
Early onset of swallowing problems
Early onset of difficulty with urinating
Blood pressure problems (fainting, lightheadedness on standing)
Symptoms and signs that mostly affect the legs
Sudden onset of symptoms

Table 10.1 lists some symptoms that suggest a diagnosis other than Parkinson's disease.

ESSENTIAL TREMOR

Many other forms of tremor exist besides that found in people who have Parkinson's disease. One, called *essential tremor*, is estimated to be the most common of all movement disorders. Also called *familial tremor*, essential tremor usually involves no other symptoms besides tremor and, unlike Parkinson's disease, it frequently runs in families. People who have essential tremor can often list parents, grandparents, siblings, or even children who have a similar tremor. Although most neurologists accept the definition that essential tremor (ET) is mono-symptomatic (postural and kinetic tremor only; that is, tremor is present when the arms are outstretched or when the person is reaching for an object), there has been recent work suggesting that ET may sometimes be linked to more extensive neurodegenerative changes. This is very controversial.

Essential tremor is actually quite distinct from the tremor seen in Parkinson's, because it is what movement disorder specialists call a *kinetic tremor*, a tremor that appears when a person's hands are moving rather than when they are still. For example, a kinetic tremor is more

Archimedes spiral: Draw between the lines from inside to outside.

Left hand   Right hand

Patient with essential tremor

Handwriting sample: Write "Today is a nice day in Baltimore."

Patient with essential tremor

Patient with Parkinson's disease

FIGURE 10.1 Tremor assessment form.

likely to be apparent when people pick up or put down a cup and sau-
cer. Their hand may shake when they are eating soup with a spoon
or when they write or draw (Figure 10.1). In Parkinson's disease, the
tremor is evident when the hand is still and is therefore called a *resting
tremor*.

Essential tremor most commonly affects the arms, although it may
also affect the head or, less commonly, the voice. When essential
tremor affects the voice, it produces a rhythmic or quivering quality that
sometimes leads other people (especially over the phone) to mistakenly
think the person has just stopped crying. The typical arm tremor starts

out mild, often in one arm but more commonly in both, and progresses very slowly over decades. People often remember that their tremor began when they were in high school or in their twenties, especially when they were under stress, and was nothing more than a curiosity or minor inconvenience for thirty or forty years or longer.

Essential tremor can cause disability. Some people find that every time they reach for a glass of water or cup of coffee, their hand shakes so uncontrollably that they spill the liquid. People usually compensate by moving tasks to the less affected side, using two hands, or sometimes even changing how they do certain activities, such as drinking soup rather than eating it with a spoon.

When essential tremor affects the head, people develop a rhythmic head shaking, either up and down as in nodding "yes" or side to side as in shaking the head to convey "no." This is distinct from any tremor of the head occurring in patients with Parkinson's disease, which is almost always limited to a tremor around the mouth involving facial muscles, jaw, or tongue. People who have Parkinson's almost never have a tremor that causes pure shaking of the head.

Alcohol has a peculiar effect on more than three-quarters of people who have essential tremor. After they drink a single glass of wine or a cocktail, their tremor is markedly improved for forty-five minutes to an hour. The effect on tremor in Parkinson's is not so dramatic.

Essential tremor also produces distinctive handwriting that in no way resembles the handwriting seen in Parkinson's disease (Figure 10.2). It is large, scrawled, and wavy, and the effect of the tremor is obvious. The handwriting of people who have Parkinson's is small and gets progressively smaller toward the end of a sentence (i.e., the more the person writes, the smaller the handwriting gets). Almost everyone who works in a movement disorder center has received letters from people written in unmistakable essential-tremor script describing how they have been diagnosed with Parkinson's disease and detailing the number of antiparkinson medications that have not helped them. From the handwriting, it is obvious that the patient does not have Parkinson's disease but essential tremor.

Potentially effective treatments for essential tremor include propranolol (Inderal) or primidone (Mysoline). In severe cases, surgical

FIGURE 10.2 Handwriting samples from patients with essential tremor.

approaches (thalamotomy or thalamic deep brain stimulation) used to treat parkinsonian tremor can also be extremely effective in treating kinetic tremor (see Chapter 16).

People who have Parkinson's sometimes have a mild kinetic tremor in addition to other physical signs of Parkinson's, so the presence of a kinetic tremor does not mean that the person definitely does not have Parkinson's disease.

The FDA in the United States recently approved dopamine imaging techniques (SPECT Scanning) as a diagnostic tool in differentiating ET from parkinsonism. The SPECT Scan (DATScan) can identify whether the dopamine system in the human brain is normal or not. In ET the dopamine system is normal and in parkinsonism, it is not. Therefore, the test could be useful to distinguish the tremor seen in ET from the tremor seen in parkinsonism. Of course, this is a distinction—resting tremor in parkinsonism and a postural or kinetic tremor in ET—which all physicians should be able to make without any specific imaging test. It is estimated that the cost of the test will be approximately $3,000 and it is unclear how this additional expenditure will benefit patients. A small proportion of people who are elderly and have ET can have some parkinsonian features, possibly due to coincidental small strokes or medications. Others can have tremor present at rest as well as with action. In these people a DATScan may be useful in helping to exclude Parkinson's disease. As discussed earlier, the DATScan cannot diagnose Parkinson's because it cannot distinguish between Parkinson's and the various cousins of Parkinson's (Parkinson's-plus, atypical parkinsonism) that exist.

HUNTINGTON'S DISEASE

Huntington's disease is a genetic disorder that usually appears between ages thirty and forty-five. The primary symptoms of this disorder in its typical form are a devastating combination of involuntary dance-like movements, called *chorea* (the Greek word for "dance"), and progressive dementia. Medical advances have produced a genetic test that can confirm whether or not a person has Huntington's. The confusion with Parkinson's disease arises in two separate situations.

First, an atypical type of Huntington's disease produces symptoms of stiffness, rigidity, and lack of movement similar to those found in Parkinson's. This type of Huntington's disease differs from Parkinson's in that tremor (especially tremor at rest) is uncommon. Also, people who have this type of Huntington's disease generally are much younger (usually under twenty) than people who have Parkinson's. Yet there is enough similarity in symptoms between the two diseases that misdiagnosis occurs.

Second, involuntary dance-like movements are one symptom of too much dopamine activity in the brain. These movements can occur when sensitivity to levodopa medications builds up in a person who has Parkinson's disease, and they can occur spontaneously in people who have Huntington's disease. If an adult has typical Huntington's chorea, with only mild mental changes, the chorea might be treated with drugs that act against the dopamine receptors. Any drug that interferes with the dopamine system, either by depleting dopamine or by blocking dopamine receptors in the brain, can produce parkinsonism that resembles Parkinson's disease. The *dopamine receptor antagonists* and the *dopamine depletor* tetrabenazine used to treat chorea in Huntington's interfere with the dopamine system and decrease dance-like movements, and these also may produce parkinsonism as a side effect. For this reason, people who have Huntington's disease who have symptoms of parkinsonism are sometimes mistaken for people who have Parkinson's. And people who have Parkinson's disease who have involuntary movements related to levodopa administration may move in a way similar to a person who has Huntington's disease.

As discussed in Chapter 9, drug-induced parkinsonism is a common problem that can be mistaken for Parkinson's disease if the history of drug treatment is not carefully scrutinized. Dopamine receptor antagonists and dopamine depletors are two classes of drugs that can cause parkinsonism.

TICS

A tic is a brief, often repetitive, involuntary movement that starts abruptly, occurs quickly, and lasts a short time. Tics can be simple or complex movements or sounds. Simple tics include shoulder shrugging, eye blinking, grunting, and sniffing. Complex tics include movements such as touching, groping, or eye blinking, followed by mouth grimacing and shoulder shrugging. Some people have a single tic all their lives; sometimes neurologists call this a *chronic motor tic*.

Gilles de la Tourette's syndrome, or simply *Tourette's syndrome*, which is thought to be genetically determined, is a well-known tic disorder. Tourette's syndrome typically involves a combination of motor and vocal tics that come and go over the years. The motor tics may involve one area of the body and then move to another. The vocal tics may consist of one sound and, later, another. Most of the vocal tics are actually nonverbal utterances, such as grunts. Although it is quite uncommon, the best-known Tourette's vocal tic, called *coprolalia,* is the involuntary utterance of swear words and profanities. The frequency and severity of the tics may vary markedly over time.

Tourette's syndrome is usually a lifelong disorder. In addition, Tourette's syndrome is often associated with obsessive-compulsive behavior, such as repeatedly checking to see whether a light has been switched off before leaving the house or repeatedly washing the hands. Tics in Tourette's syndrome can be controlled with a wide variety of drugs. There is usually no difficulty in distinguishing tic disorders from Parkinson's disease, although a repetitive movement might be mistaken for a tremor. As mentioned in the section on Huntington's disease, drugs that antagonize the effects of dopamine, which are also commonly used to treat tics, may cause drug-induced parkinsonism.

TYPES OF DYSTONIA

Used literally, the word *dystonia* refers to any abnormal muscle tone, whether too limp or too tense. However, in clinical usage, *dystonia* is a type of movement disorder characterized by muscle spasm that causes sustained twisting postures. Dystonia can occur by itself or in the setting of a number of neurologic disorders. Parkinson's itself sometimes produces dystonia that appears as foot and occasionally hand cramping (see Chapter 3).

Another dystonia appears most often in persons under the age of twenty. This disabling and progressive disorder involves abnormal movements of the legs or arms or both, consisting of slow, twisting, writhing movements, usually with sustained abnormal postures.

When dystonia first appears in adults, it tends to be focused in one or two related areas of the body. This is referred to as *focal* or *segmental dystonia*. Writer's cramp is an example of a focal dystonia that is specific to a particular task. A person's hand is perfectly functional except during the act of handwriting, when his or her hand twists and turns into an abnormal, at times painful, posture that prevents writing. *Spasmodic torticollis (cervical dystonia)* is another focal dystonia in which the head and neck are rotated, tilted, flexed forward, or extended backward. *Lower limb dystonia* in adults usually involves the turning inward of the foot with curling of the toes. This can be painful and interfere with walking.

Types of dystonia affecting the face include *blepharospasm* and *oromandibular dystonia*. In blepharospasm, the eyelids involuntarily close intermittently. Because the eyes cannot be opened at will, this kind of dystonia may cause functional blindness or other visual impairment. In oromandibular dystonia, the jaw closes or opens involuntarily and the face may twist or contort into grimaces.

Another dystonia, which may be inherited, is called *levodopa-responsive dystonia* or *dopa-responsive dystonia* (DRD). Caused by a specific enzyme defect in the brain's dopamine system, this type of dystonia usually begins in the leg and often spreads to involve the rest of the body. In about 75 percent of people it affects, this dystonia has the peculiar property of varying in intensity throughout the day, sometimes quite markedly. Affected children may have times of the day when they have almost no neurologic abnormality (e.g., in the morning or after a nap) and other times (e.g., later in the day or after exercise) when they are unable to walk because of the prominent twisted posture of a foot or leg. The administration of carbidopa/levodopa in extremely low doses dramatically improves the dystonia of DRD. Parkinsonism may be seen with DRD, occasionally in children and more often in adults; nonetheless, DRD is distinct from Parkinson's disease.

The dystonia that occurs with Parkinson's sometimes causes diagnostic confusion. Very rarely, probably in less than 1 percent of people who have Parkinson's, dystonia is the initial symptom of Parkinson's disease. Dystonia early on, unrelated to antiparkinson medication, is more common in young-onset Parkinson's. In Chapter 4 we described the relatively common dystonia of the feet or hands in moderate to advanced Parkinson's disease. People's big toe may bend up and press against their shoe, they may have painful cramping, their fingers may curl up, their thumb may move to an awkward position, their foot may turn in, or their toes fan out. Given these symptoms, a neurologist is likely to believe initially that the problem is an isolated dystonia, until a thorough examination reveals subtle evidence of emerging Parkinson's symptoms. The drugs used to treat Parkinson's (especially levodopa and dopamine agonists) may also induce various forms of dystonia. There are a variety of other relatively uncommon neurological diseases in which dystonia and parkinsonism co-occur, often in younger individuals. Diagnosis can often be very challenging although MRI and selected genetic testing can sometimes provide an accurate diagnosis.

WILSON'S DISEASE

Accurate diagnosis for a person who has Wilson's disease is vital, because treatment can prevent neurologic abnormalities and a potentially fatal outcome. Wilson's disease is an extremely rare genetic disease that can have many of the same symptoms as Parkinson's, but Wilson's disease, unlike Parkinson's disease, can be diagnosed with a simple test.

Wilson's is caused by an abnormality of copper metabolism that deposits excessive copper in the liver, brain, eyes, and kidneys. The symptoms of Wilson's disease usually begin before the age of twenty-five. The most common age for liver-predominant Wilson's disease to emerge is around twelve to fourteen. Neurologic symptoms often begin in late adolescence.

The neurologic symptoms of Wilson's disease include tremors, slowness, and clumsiness of movement, gait difficulty, and emotional problems. People under the age of twenty or twenty-five who appear to have the symptoms of Parkinson's disease might have Wilson's disease instead. The symptoms can be similar, but the young age of the patient is a clue that this is not typical Parkinson's.

The main obstacle to diagnosing Wilson's disease is its rarity. Many physicians never see a person who has Wilson's disease. Although most people who have Wilson's seek the help of a physician before age twenty-five, the disease can also appear at a later age. We teach our medical students and neurology residents that any person under the age of forty-five who develops an unusual neurologic problem that involves tremor, slowness of movement, dystonia, rigidity, or gait difficulty should be evaluated for Wilson's disease. Because people who have Wilson's are usually much younger than those with Parkinson's, confusion is not common.

If you have symptoms of Parkinson's and are in your thirties, you may wish to ask your doctor if there is any possibility that you have Wilson's disease.

PARKINSON'S-PLUS SYNDROMES

As noted in Chapter 8, the cluster of symptoms characteristic of Parkinson's disease is commonly seen in a number of related neurodegenerative disorders, called *Parkinson's-plus,* or *atypical Parkinson's.* These various disorders often cause diagnostic confusion. Many people who have these symptoms believe they have Parkinson's, but they actually have one of the other types of parkinsonism.

The underlying changes in the brain in Parkinson's-plus disorders are different from the changes seen in Parkinson's. This means that the Parkinson's-plus syndromes may appear at different ages, produce different types of disabilities, and vary in the speed with which problems become apparent. Medications effective in Parkinson's disease are generally less effective or ineffective in atypical Parkinson's. An accurate diagnosis is crucial so that the course of a person's disease can be assessed and the appropriate treatment recommended.

Physicians can't always tell early in the disease which of the many "cousins" of Parkinson's disease a person has, but with time, certain distinctive features of each syndrome will appear and help differentiate these disorders from Parkinson's. Although there is a debate among neurologists about the fine points of discriminating between syndromes, in this section we identify some key features that may help the patient or family distinguish between typical Parkinson's and one of its "cousins."

Some Parkinson's-plus disorders, such as multiple system atrophy (MSA) and progressive supranuclear palsy (PSP), are more common than others. Other important causes of parkinsonism are dementia with Lewy bodies, corticobasal degeneration (CBD), and Alzheimer's disease. In Alzheimer's disease, cognitive impairment is the major and dominant symptom, with motor symptoms appearing later in the course of illness.

Multiple System Atrophy (MSA)

Multiple system atrophy comprises three subgroups previously believed to be distinct diseases known as *Shy-Drager syndrome, striatonigral degeneration,* and *olivopontocerebellar degeneration.* In Shy-Drager syndrome, the autonomic nervous system does not function well, producing urinary, sexual function, and blood pressure symptoms in addition to the rigidity, slowness, and gait difficulties of parkinsonism. When the autonomic nervous system is severely impaired, people may feel the need to urinate frequently or with great urgency, or they may become incontinent. Males may have difficulty achieving a sexual erection. (Little research has been done on the effects on female sexual response.) When the autonomic reflex that controls blood pressure is impaired, people find that when they stand up suddenly, their blood pressure falls so low that they become lightheaded, dizzy, sweaty, and weak. Their vision blurs and they may even faint. This symptom, called *orthostatic hypotension*, is relieved when the person lies down or lowers his or her head. If these autonomic nervous system symptoms appear early in the course of the disorder, it is wise to suspect Shy-Drager syndrome (now referred to by the all encompassing term, multiple system atrophy or MSA) rather than Parkinson's.

People who have the striatonigral degeneration form of MSA have progressive parkinsonism characterized by rigidity, slowness, gait difficulties, and possibly tremor, but they rarely respond to antiparkinson medications as expected. Especially in the early years of this form of MSA (often referred to as MSA-P emphasizing the dominant feature of parkinsonism), it may be impossible to differentiate the clinical features from typical Parkinson's disease.

In olivopontocerebellar degeneration, unlike in Parkinson's disease, the cerebellum is also affected (resulting in the term MSA-C for this variant). People who have this disorder have a different type of clumsiness, slurred speech, and gait disturbance in addition to the parkinsonian syndrome. The differences between olivopontocerebellar degeneration and Parkinson's are subtle. If your Parkinson's symptoms seem a little odd, it might be useful to see a movement disorder neurologist.

These three "separate" syndromes were recognized as part of a spectrum of neurodegeneration and the term MSA was used to describe the entire group. With the advancement of basic research, we have now recognized that MSA is part of a neurodegeneration process that somehow involves the same protein involved in Parkinson's disease, α synuclein. Alpha synuclein accumulates and aggregates in a different fashion in the two disorders and how it contributes to the neurodegeneration in both remains unknown. Given the similarity in the abnormal protein accumulation in Parkinson's and MSA these are now sometimes called synucleinopathies.

When Parkinson's disease drugs are used that replace, mimic, or stimulate the missing dopamine, people who have any of the three subtypes of MSA don't respond as well as would be expected if they had Parkinson's. If a person who has symptoms of parkinsonism experiences only very slight symptomatic relief from antiparkinson medications, the value of continuing the medication should be carefully considered under the supervision of the neurologist.

Progressive Supranuclear Palsy (PSP)

The primary symptom of progressive supranuclear palsy is difficulty with eye movement, particularly moving eyes up or down. People who have PSP may be unable to see food on their plate or to notice an obstacle in their path when walking. Some have a tremor, although this is not a predominant element of their illness.

People who have PSP also typically have the parkinsonian syndrome of rigidity, slowness of movement, and severe gait and balance problems. Gait and balance problems are more prominent symptoms in PSP, are more severe, and appear earlier than in Parkinson's disease. If someone begins to experience early difficulties with falling, this is an important clue that the problem may be PSP.

People who have PSP sometimes respond well to antiparkinson medication for a brief time, but these medications are less effective in treating PSP than true Parkinson's disease.

The abnormal protein in PSP that accumulates is called TAU. The TAU protein is seen not only in PSP, but also in CBD (and a number of other disorders usually causing forms of dementia) and these Parkinson's-plus syndromes are now known as tauopathies.

Corticobasal Degeneration (CBD)

People who have corticobasal degeneration can experience a wide array of symptoms. Typically the symptoms are asymmetric, with one side of the body much more affected than the other. In addition to parkinsonism, the person has difficulty with voluntary movement beyond that explained by akinesia. *Apraxia* results in both profound clumsiness and apparent difficulties knowing *how* to perform complex movements. The person who has CBD may also have jerky movement (myoclonus) that is sometimes mistaken for tremor. Dystonia of the limb may be profound. Some individuals have an unusual symptom known as the *alien limb phenomenon* in which a limb (usually the hand) spontaneously performs activities they do not wish it to do. Finally, behavioral, language, and cognitive changes are common in CBD, and some people experience these problems early in the course of the disease. Just as the term parkinsonism refers to a Parkinson's disease–like syndrome caused by various diseases, the term "corticobasal syndrome" (CBS) is now being used to highlight the fact that several different brain diseases can cause the same clinical picture that was first described due to CBD.

Other Disorders with Parkinsonism

For people who have a number of other disorders, early cognitive (mental) and personality changes may be accompanied or followed by symptoms of mild parkinsonism, such as a slight intermittent resting tremor, slight slowness of movement, or slight shuffling with loss of balance. Their most prominent symptoms may be difficulty with memory, personality changes, and difficulty concentrating. For example, they may have problems remembering to attend to everyday financial matters or remembering the shopping list when they go to the store. People who have these disorders may also have visual hallucinations and delusions that are not provoked by medication but instead are symptoms of the underlying illness itself.

When such personality or memory changes or thinking problems develop within the first few years of the onset of the parkinsonian motor symptoms, the correct diagnosis is unlikely to be typical Parkinson's disease. The person may have Alzheimer's disease complicated by parkinsonian features or another parkinsonian syndrome called dementia with Lewy bodies (or diffuse Lewy body disease). Dementia with Lewy bodies (DLB) is a relative of Parkinson's disease. The hallmark feature of Parkinson's, the Lewy body (see Chapter 1) is present in both and indeed, at autopsy the brain pathology is often indistinguishable from that found in Parkinson's patients who experienced dementia later in the course. In fact, many believe that there is a spectrum that exists between these disorders rather than considering them distinct and separate entities. It is likely that important breakthroughs in management of one of these will have clear implications for the other.

Dementia may also be caused by a treatable condition unrelated to the symptoms of parkinsonism, and laboratory tests can identify some of these illnesses. These tests include a routine complete blood count and evaluations of thyroid function, vitamin B_{12} and folate levels, and sedimentation rate. A test for syphilis should also be considered. Such tests are important in identifying treatable conditions that are associated with cognitive impairment, such as low thyroid function.

Neuroimaging studies such as a computerized axial tomography (CAT) scan or magnetic resonance imaging (MRI) of the brain may also uncover unusual but potentially treatable causes of dementia, such as normal-pressure hydrocephalus, subdural hematoma, benign or malignant brain tumors, or the silent strokes discussed in Chapter 9.

IN SOME PEOPLE, several years may pass before the more distinctive features of one of the "cousins" of Parkinson's disease emerge, and at that point a Parkinson's diagnosis may need to be changed. Because of the wide variety of neurologic disorders that must be considered when parkinsonian symptoms appear, we advise patients and their families to see an expert in the treatment of neurologic disease to help them arrive at a correct diagnosis and proper plan of treatment.

Part IV

TREATMENT OF PARKINSON'S DISEASE

CHAPTER 11

How the Brain Works and How Treatment Works

- *How does Parkinson's affect the brain and nervous system?*
- *How does this relate to symptoms?*
- *How do medications work to overcome these problems?*

Although Parkinson's disease affects the function of the muscles and may appear to be a disease of the muscles, the muscles themselves are not the problem. The difficulty lies in the complex system that transfers the *idea of a movement,* which occurs in the brain, to the *actual movement,* in the muscle. To explain how Parkinson's affects a person and how it can be treated, we need to consider the workings of the brain and nervous system.

THE MOTOR CONTROL SYSTEM

The basic outline of motor control is as follows. Let's say you decide—a process occurring in your brain—to bend your fingers to make a fist. In order to carry out this task, a signal for the task is relayed along a series of nerve cells, called *neurons,* in the brain and spinal cord, all the way down to the muscles in the hand. Signals are relayed from one neuron to another along the neuron's long fiber, called the *axon.* At the end of the axon, the signal flashes across a space between the cells called the *synaptic cleft* (Figure 11.1). The signal then activates the next cell, which carries it along the axon to the next cell, which carries

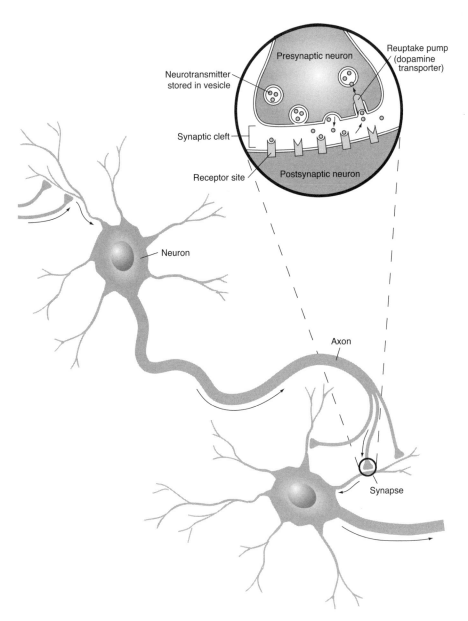

FIGURE 11.1 This figure illustrates how neurons communicate with each other. The drawing shows neurons and their nerve fibers connecting to other neurons. These connections are called *synapses*. The blowup of the synapse in the *top of the figure* shows some of the essential cellular machinery that is involved in transmitting messages from one neuron to another.

the signal along—and so on. When the signal reaches the hand, the muscles contract on the palm side of the fingers, and you make a fist.

Until relatively recently, how neurons signal each other across the synaptic cleft was a great mystery. We now know that when the signal reaches the end of the axon, it activates release of a biological chemical, a *neurotransmitter*, which transmits neural signals. The neurotransmitter flashes across the synaptic cleft to specialized receptor sites on an adjacent neuron. The neurotransmitter is picked up by the adjacent neuron, the signal travels along that neuron's axon, and the process is then repeated—and all of this happens amazingly quickly.

There you have it: The signal passes along the neuron to the end of its axon, where a neurotransmitter is released and crosses the synaptic cleft to the receptors on the next neuron, and so on and so on, until the muscle contracts. Of course, the process isn't that simple. The signal doesn't simply travel from a thought center directly to the fingers—it has to be modulated on the way. And this modulation takes place in the brain.

The brain is divided into three main sections: the two cerebral hemispheres (together known as the *cerebrum*), the *cerebellum*, and the *brain stem*. At the base of the brain are two large groups of nerve cells called the *basal ganglia*, which are made up of the *putamen*, the *caudate*, and the *globus pallidus* (Figure 11.2). The putamen and caudate together make up the *striatum*. The basal ganglia are intricately connected with almost all other regions of the brain, and they play a large role in modulating signals for normal and abnormal motor activity. The caudate, the putamen, and the globus pallidus form part of the circuit that is not functioning properly in Parkinson's disease.

The brain's signal to the muscles first travels from the *cerebral cortex* (the outer surface of the cerebrum) to the basal ganglia and other brain structures, which are thought to accept the signals from the cortex and then modify them. These modified signals pass into another brain structure called the *thalamus* and back to the cerebral cortex. Information is modified by intricate, reverberating loops and connections. All this modulation and functioning is made possible by neurotransmitters. When the signal has been appropriately modulated, an output signal from the thalamus goes back to the thinking cortex, and the motor signal finally gets sent out.

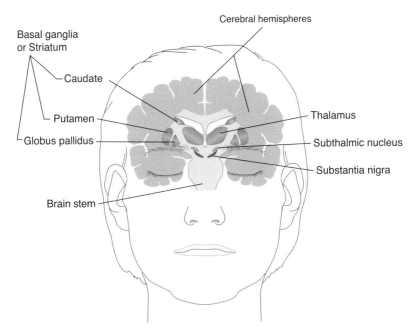

FIGURE 11.2 This figure illustrates various structures that are important in normal motor control, as well as the location of these structures in relation to one other.

There are at least fifteen different neurotransmitters, including dopamine, acetylcholine, norepinephrine (also called noradrenaline), serotonin, and glutamate. Each has different, specific, necessary functions. Some neurotransmitters open certain "gates" in membranes so that a signal can go through; some close other gates to funnel the signal in another direction. A delicate balance exists between all these systems. An imbalance between these systems results in disruption of the signal from the brain to the muscles, causing tremor, rigidity, and slowness of movement. The dopaminergic system is the most important player in the functioning of the basal ganglia.

What Happens in Parkinson's Disease

The symptoms noted above—tremor, rigidity, slowness—are the TRAP symptoms of Parkinson's disease. When symptoms of parkinsonism appear, they invariably involve problems with the dopaminergic system and, in Parkinson's disease, the substantia nigra and basal ganglia. As noted in Chapter 1, the substantia nigra is a very small area located deep within the brain (there are actually two structures, but they are generally referred to as a single entity in the medical literature).

The substantia nigra is full of dopamine-producing cells, which deliver their product (dopamine) to the basal ganglia and other parts of the brain. Because this path for motor control includes both the substantia nigra and the striatum, it is called the *nigrostriatal pathway*. When the substantia nigra is damaged and the dopamine cells malfunction, the dopamine supply to the caudate and putamen (the striatum) is gradually reduced until, eventually, the symptoms of Parkinson's disease emerge—generally when about 50 percent of the cells in the substantia nigra are damaged.

When the dopamine-relayed messages to the striatum and other motor centers are disrupted, the delicate balancing act of neurochemical systems is disturbed, resulting in the motor symptoms of Parkinson's disease. Parkinson's is not just a dopamine deficiency state, however. Less prominent, secondary neurotransmitter and cell changes throughout the brain cause symptoms, too. In Parkinson's, other small nuclear centers within the brain (e.g., the *dorsal motor nucleus of the vagus* and the *locus ceruleus*) also are affected by the degeneration. The brain concentrations of other transmitters, such as norepinephrine and serotonin, are also altered.

HOW DOES MEDICATION THERAPY WORK?

In Chapters 12 and 13 we discuss specific medications in detail. Here we want to concentrate on describing *how* these medications work, given what we know about how the brain functions normally and how it is affected in Parkinson's disease.

Anticholinergics

Following James Parkinson's first description of Parkinson's disease in 1817, efforts were begun to find an effective treatment. Between 1860 and 1870, belladonna alkaloids (now known as *anticholinergic* medications) were first introduced for the treatment of Parkinson's disease in the clinic of the famous French neurologist Jean-Martin Charcot. The belladonna alkaloids were found to be effective for many disorders, including the "shaking palsy." Anticholinergic agents originally were developed from the herb belladonna. Although belladonna could be hazardous, it was widely used by women at the royal courts of Europe as an infusion to make the pupils of their eyes larger and thus, it was thought, more beautiful (*bella*). Doctors observed that people using belladonna experienced a dry mouth, and they began prescribing belladonna to control drooling in people who have Parkinson's. They soon found out, however, that the drug also decreased the tremor.

Anticholinergic agents affect one of the most common neurotransmitters in the brain, acetylcholine. Disruption of the balance between the effects of dopamine and the effects of acetylcholine in the basal ganglia contributes to the clinical symptoms of Parkinson's disease. The belladonna alkaloids reduce cholinergic activity and in that way help to reset the balance between dopamine and acetylcholine in the brain. Parkinson's depletes dopamine, leaving the cholinergic system with a larger than normal role in the intricate loops and circuits of muscle signals and control. When the anticholinergics block the cholinergic system, some balance between the two systems is reestablished.

The benefit of using anticholinergics to treat Parkinson's disease is primarily in reducing the resting tremor. These drugs have substantial side effects, but by starting at low doses and managing them carefully, many patients have found them beneficial. Their use in older people, especially those with preexisting thinking and memory problems, is largely contraindicated.

Levodopa

Levodopa remains the mainstay of therapy for people who have Parkinson's disease. It has been in widespread use since the late 1960s. The discovery of levodopa's effectiveness in the treatment of Parkinson's disease is remarkable to this day and illustrates many facets of both neuroscience research and clinical research.

Until the late 1950s, levodopa and dopamine were thought to be simply the products of intermediate steps in the formation of the neurotransmitter norepinephrine (noradrenaline). Almost all the focus of neuroscience research during this era was directed at understanding more about norepinephrine.

Only when researchers began to examine regional concentrations of different chemicals within the brain did unexpected findings begin to appear. While examining how much of one chemical was in one part of the brain and how much was in another, researchers made the unexpected discovery of very high concentrations of levodopa and dopamine in the basal ganglia, particularly in the caudate and putamen. High dopamine concentrations in these regions would not be expected if dopamine were simply a metabolic stepping-stone in the pathway from levodopa to norepinephrine. Then in the late 1950s and early 1960s, researchers discovered that the concentration of dopamine was very *low* in the caudate and putamen in autopsy specimens from people who have Parkinson's disease. This was the first time that a specific neurodegenerative disease could be linked with a specific chemical deficiency, namely dopamine, in a specific region of the brain, the caudate and putamen.

When researchers discovered that the shortage of dopamine was associated with Parkinson's symptoms, the obvious course was to administer dopamine to people who have Parkinson's disease. This strategy, however, did not work.

To keep out materials that could be damaging to brain cells, the brain has a protective mechanism called the *blood-brain barrier*. This barrier contains a layer of specialized cells that prevents certain types of substances from directly entering the brain from the bloodstream. One of those substances is dopamine, which therefore cannot cross the blood-brain barrier. Consequently, orally administered dopamine is not helpful in treating Parkinson's because it does not reach the brain, where it is needed. Confronted with this obstacle to replacing dopamine in the brain, researchers looked about for the next most logical candidate.

As shown in Figure 11.3, levodopa is the immediately preceding chemical, or *precursor,* from which dopamine is made. (A precursor is a chemical that can be metabolized into another chemical.) Levodopa *does* cross the blood-brain barrier and is converted to dopamine within the brain, as well as elsewhere in the body. This chemical reaction, like all chemical reactions in living tissues, is controlled by an enzyme. Levodopa is converted to dopamine by way of the enzyme *dopa decarboxylase.* (The role of dopa decarboxylase is discussed later.)

Levodopa was first given to people who have Parkinson's disease in the early 1960s, with mixed results. The debate about its usefulness for treating Parkinson's began. Some reports claimed that levodopa alleviated certain symptoms; others indicated that levodopa was of no use for Parkinson's. The debate continued until the late 1960s, when Dr. George Cotzias, working with his colleagues in New York, reported that when large doses of levodopa were administered orally, patients experienced a dramatic improvement of the symptoms of Parkinson's disease. The news was nothing short of startling. Films of people who had been in wheelchairs and were now playing baseball were shown on television news programs across America.

This was a dramatic breakthrough in the therapy of a neurodegenerative disorder, and it was very large doses of levodopa that did it. During the previous eight or nine years, investigators had been administering 100 to 300 milligrams of levodopa, but Dr. Cotzias and his colleagues administered 3,000 to 5,000 milligrams. (The story of the spectacular

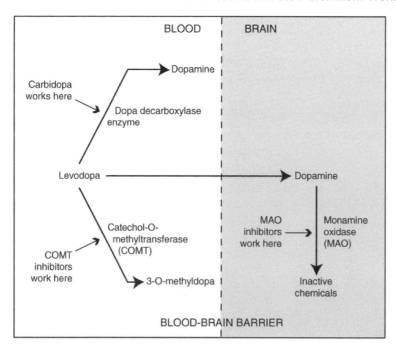

FIGURE 11.3 This figure illustrates how levodopa crosses the blood-brain barrier and enters the brain and becomes (is metabolized into) dopamine. The figure also demonstrates that outside the blood-brain barrier there are two enzymes, dopa decarboxylase and catechol-O-methyltransferase (COMT), that degrade levodopa and decrease its effectiveness. Carbidopa, which is a component of carbidopa/levodopa, and the COMT inhibitors (entacapone [Comtan] and tolcapone [Tasmar]) inhibit these enzymes and allow levodopa to more readily enter the brain to be converted to dopamine. Within the brain, MAO inhibitors (selegiline, rasagiline) slow the destruction of dopamine; thus, more dopamine is available.

successes with levodopa appeared in a slightly different setting in Oliver Sacks's book *Awakenings* and in the movie of the same name.)

New discoveries tied dopamine to motor function. Swedish scientists were able to demonstrate for the first time that dopamine-producing cells are present in the substantia nigra and that these cells deliver dopamine to the caudate and putamen. It became clear that this pathway is fundamental to normal motor function and that when the substantia nigra is damaged and the dopamine-producing cells malfunction, the dopamine supply to the caudate and putamen is gradually reduced until the symptoms of Parkinson's disease emerge. This discovery tied together brain anatomy, biochemistry, and treatment, and it formed the basis of our understanding of Parkinson's disease. (Dr. Arvid Carlsson won the Nobel Prize for work in this field in 2000.)

Dopa Decarboxylase Inhibitors (DDIs)

Levodopa was not perfect, however. Dopa decarboxylase, the enzyme that converts levodopa to dopamine, is also found in places outside the brain—the gastrointestinal tract, kidneys, liver, and other regions of the body. Outside the brain, dopa decarboxylase snatches up the administered levodopa and converts it to dopamine before it can get past the blood-brain barrier. This process not only keeps the levodopa from reaching the brain, it also produces large quantities of dopamine in the bloodstream. This high dopamine level is particularly known for stimulating nausea and vomiting; rarely, it causes a drop in blood pressure and changes in heart rhythm.

A solution to the problem of gastrointestinal upset was to stop the enzyme from hijacking levodopa in other regions of the body so that the levodopa would be fully available in the brain. Researchers developed *peripheral dopa decarboxylase inhibitors,* or DDIs. (Here, *peripheral* means that these drugs act outside the blood-brain barrier.) In the digestive tract and other areas of the body, DDIs block the enzyme's conversion of levodopa to dopamine. This permits more of the administered levodopa to travel to the brain unaltered. Once there, because the DDIs are excluded from the brain, dopa decarboxylase within the brain converts levodopa to dopamine. The required dosage of levodopa combined with a DDI is much lower than the dosage of levodopa alone, yet it still produces the desired beneficial effect. Before the use of DDIs, levodopa dosages might reach 4,000 to 6,000 milligrams per day (as first used by George Cotzias). With DDIs, a therapeutic dosage of levodopa ranges from 150 to 1,500 milligrams per day. Nausea and vomiting are markedly reduced. Today, levodopa is available only in combination tablets containing a DDI. In the United States, the only DDI available is carbidopa; elsewhere, benserazide is also available. Sometimes, when the amount of DDI combined with levodopa is inadequate and gastrointestinal side effects persist (typically, early in treatment), additional separate carbidopa can be useful.

Another way of treating the side effects of dopamine caused by its effects outside the brain is with a dopamine receptor blocker that works exclusively outside the brain (and therefore does not cause worsening of Parkinson's disease, as occurs with typical and some atypical neuroleptics). Domperidone is one such drug. It can also be effective for treating similar side effects occurring with dopamine receptor agonists (see below). DDIs are not useful here, since these drugs do not require metabolism by dopa decarboxylase to exert their effects.

Dopamine Receptor Agonists

There is yet another complication, however. Parkinson's involves the degeneration of cells that produce dopamine, yet levodopa therapy requires those same cells to convert levodopa to dopamine. As Parkinson's disease becomes more advanced, this conversion process becomes sluggish. Other cells pick up the slack, but they do not exercise the same subtle regulation as do the cells of the substantia nigra.

Researchers therefore had to come up with a new approach. As described earlier, a neurotransmitter is released from one axon and flashes across the synaptic cleft to its specific receptor on an adjacent neuron, which then takes up the signal and passes it on. The new scheme that researchers developed uses synthetic drugs to stimulate the receptors just as dopamine does. A drug capable of combining with receptors to imitate the action of a neurotransmitter is called an *agonist*. (An *antagonist* would neutralize, or impede, the action of the neurotransmitter; the neuroleptics we discussed earlier [in Chapter 9], capable of causing drug-induced parkinsonism, do so by blocking dopamine receptors—i.e., they are dopamine receptor antagonists.) A dopamine receptor agonist, then, mimics the activity of dopamine at the dopamine receptor, stimulates the transmission of nerve signals, and thereby relieves symptoms of Parkinson's.

Researchers have developed a number of dopamine receptor agonists. The brain has at least five types of dopamine receptors, denoted by D_1, D_2, D_3, D_4, and D_5. Each of the dopamine receptors has distinct properties, and we still have much to learn about them. To be effective in treating the characteristic symptoms of Parkinson's disease, agonists must stimulate the D_2 receptor. (Chapter 13 and Figure 13.1 provide more detail about this process.)

COMT (Catechol-O-Methyltransferase) Inhibitors

Another enzyme that hijacks levodopa medication and converts it to a chemical that does not cross the blood-brain barrier is catechol-O-methyltransferase (COMT). Inhibitors of this enzyme, the COMT inhibitors, prevent the conversion of levodopa and therefore operate on almost exactly the same principle as DDIs. Usually the dose of levodopa can be reduced further if a COMT inhibitor is added to the DDI/levodopa regimen, and COMT inhibitors are particularly helpful for people who have motor fluctuations (see Chapter 12). Entacapone and tolcapone are the two COMT inhibitors in general use. Tolcapone's use is limited by the fact that it can, rarely, induce liver malfunction.

If you are taking a COMT inhibitor, be sure to talk to your doctor about side effects and the potential need for periodic blood monitoring.

Monoamine Oxidase (MAO) Inhibitors

Just as the body has enzymes that break down levodopa, it also has enzymes that break down dopamine itself. One such enzyme is mono-amine oxidase (MAO). As discussed in Chapter 13, MAO has two subtypes, A and B. Nonselective MAO inhibitors (i.e., those that in-hibit both subtypes) and MAO-A inhibitors are used in the treatment of depression. The nonselective MAO inhibitors are dangerous and contraindicated for people taking levodopa, because this combination causes severe increases in blood pressure (the "cheese effect"). Se-lective MAO-B inhibitors, however, are useful in treating Parkinson's disease, especially when they are combined with levodopa, because they prevent some of the dopamine from being destroyed. Selegiline and rasagiline are selective MAO-B inhibitors that prevent MAO from breaking down dopamine and thus make more dopamine available in the brain.

Despite conjecture that selegiline might protect neurons from de-generation, there is no evidence that selegiline provides such protec-tion. In fact, all of selegiline's antiparkinson functions are very mild, and sometimes people cannot tell whether it has any effect at all. Rasagiline is a newer MAO-B inhibitor that has proved helpful in the symptomatic treatment of both early and more advanced Parkinson's. Selegiline and rasagiline seem to have similar effects, and there is no evidence that one is better than the other.

Although rasagiline has proven efficacy in the symptomatic treatment of Parkinson's, a recent large clinical research trial (known as the ADAGIO trial) was conducted to determine if rasagiline actively modifies or slows down the progression of Parkinson's. This trial was designed as a "delayed start" trial, which is a new type of clinical trial designed to overcome the problem of determining whether a drug that improves symptoms in Parkinson's can at the same time slow the progression of Parkinson's. In other words, can a drug have both a symptomatic effect and a neuroprotective effect?

In a typical clinical research trial, two groups of similar patients are randomized to either an active medication or placebo and are followed for a set period (e.g., six to nine months) and then are compared to see if the active medication is measurably better than the placebo. In a "delayed start trial" the patient groups are also randomized to placebo and active medication, but after a fixed time (e.g., nine months) all patients are switched to active medication and after another fixed time (e.g., nine months), the two groups are compared (see Figures 11.4 and 11.5). The main hypothesis of the delayed start trial is that if a medication is purely symptomatic, the response of the group receiving the "delayed" medication will be the same as if they had started medication from the beginning. On the other hand, if the medication is disease modifying or neuroprotective, the group that starts medication later will never "catch up" symptomatically.

The large delayed start rasagiline trial in early Parkinson's provided somewhat controversial results. One dose (2 mg per day) failed to show benefit while a second (1 mg per day) did show the desired changes, although the difference between the active and placebo groups was very small. Some researchers have interpreted the minimally statistically positive results in a favorable light. Others have examined the same results and concluded that despite a well-designed trial, the results are clinically meaningless—for example, the scale used to determine if rasagiline had an effect on neuroprotection had 176 clinical points, and the positive outcome that was statistically significant was a difference of 1.8 points or approximately a 1 percent change. Many experienced clinical research investigators determined that this was not a "clinically important" change. Unfortunately, there remains no proven neuroprotective medications in Parkinson's. An FDA advisory panel voted 17 to 0 that the results of the delayed start trial did not provide evidence of neuroprotection or disease modification.

THE BRAIN'S MOTOR CONTROL SYSTEM is marvelously complex. Sometimes when we attempt to restore it through medication, we get unwanted side effects. Many more therapies, drugs, and drug combinations are now available to alleviate and improve the symptoms of

Placebo-Controlled Clinical Trial
Mechanism unclear:
All symptomatic effect <u>or</u>
Combined symptomatic plus disease modifying?

FIGURE 11.4 A placebo-controlled clinical trial of a drug that has some effects on symptoms. Both arms show initial symptomatic improvement; the placebo group's is modest (the placebo effect) and shown here to be unsustained while the active treatment has a more marked benefit and patients remain better at the end of the trial than they were at trial onset (note the different level of symptom severity at the *end of the solid arrow line and the baseline*). At the end of the trial there is a clear difference between the placebo arm and the active drug arm (*vertical two-headed arrow*) but one cannot tell if this is entirely due to the persistent symptomatic effects of the drug or a combination of this and additional disease-modifying effects. If the treatment period is followed by a drug washout period (i.e., the treatments are withdrawn as shown here) and those receiving the active treatment don't go back to the same severity as the placebo-treated patients (*the bracket at the right side of the two solid lines*), this suggests a persistent disease-modifying effect. However, the duration of the washout must be long enough to allow all the symptomatic effects of the active drug to wear off, and these effects are often very poorly understood and may be surprisingly long-lived.

FIGURE 11.5 The delayed start design tries to address the problems of the two-arm randomized controlled clinical trial shown in Figure 11.4 (in which a withdrawal phase is not included or is not sustained long enough to answer whether the active drug is truly disease modifying). Here patients are initially randomized to placebo or active treatment, as in the earlier design. At a designated time (e.g., nine months), rather than withdrawing both drugs, the placebo treated patients are switched to the active treatment. If the effects of the active treatment are exclusively symptomatic, then the placebo group catches up and there is no difference between the two groups at the end of the study (*top graph*). However, if the active drug does have disease-modifying effects, the group receiving the active treatment initially has an important time advantage over those initially receiving the placebo, and this latter group does not catch up to those initially receiving the active treatment (*vertical two headed arrow; bottom graph*).

Parkinson's and minimize the side effects than in the past. Yet the drug regimens are themselves complex, as you will find in Chapter 13. If you are taking or planning to take medications for Parkinson's disease, understanding the possibilities will help you make decisions about your treatment plan in conjunction with people who have expertise with these therapies.

CHAPTER 12

Choosing the
Correct Medications

- *How effective are antiparkinson drugs at relieving symptoms?*
- *What about side effects from the medications?*
- *When should the drugs be started?*
- *How much medication is appropriate?*
- *Are there any proven neuroprotective medications?*

Many approaches are available for achieving the proper balance of antiparkinson medication—treating symptoms effectively while minimizing unpleasant side effects. In this chapter we discuss the considerations that go into choosing which medications to take and when to take them, and how to determine whether the drug therapy is working and when it's time for a change. We also describe medication side effects and what can be done about them. We discuss antiparkinson drugs in detail in Chapter 13: what each drug is used for, how the drugs work, and other information that people taking these drugs need to know.

As we discuss in this chapter, many issues must be considered when making medication decisions. For various reasons, many people prefer to take as little medication as possible, as late in the disease as possible, and most doctors prefer to prescribe the least amount of medication necessary. These are not always the best or most appropriate approaches; all too often we see patients who have tolerated far too much disability unnecessarily due to their poorly informed desire to delay treatment or to a well-meaning but inexperienced physician's choice to minimize their therapy. When medical research finds medications that can protect the neurologic system, it will be quite a different story: our primary goal then will become the earliest possible detection of Parkinson's disease and starting neuroprotective medication as soon as possible.

The most commonly used and most effective drug in our armamentarium against Parkinson's symptoms is *levodopa*; it is used with another drug, *carbidopa* (in other countries an alternative to carbidopa is *benserazide*), which protects levodopa from being converted to dopamine before it reaches the brain (see Chapter 11). For now, most Parkinson's disease experts agree that people who have Parkinson's need carbidopa/levodopa only when the Parkinson's motor symptoms become severe enough to impair their daily function or quality of life, whether that means recreational or job-related activities.

THERAPY MUST BE INDIVIDUALLY TAILORED

Every person who has Parkinson's disease needs to follow a program of drug therapy specifically designed for that individual. There are many reasons why this is so—why a standard regimen of medications cannot be applied across the board to everyone with Parkinson's disease.

First, in different people, different symptoms are prominent. Someone with predominant tremor may require tremor medications, while someone with considerable slowness and minimal tremor may benefit from a different medical regimen.

Second, people differ in their emotional reactions to the same symptom. Tremor might not bother one person very much, but for another person it may be very distressing or embarrassing—so much so that he or she won't leave home unless medications can relieve the tremor. One person may be able to cope with the involuntary dyskinetic movements sometimes caused by antiparkinson drugs that control motor symptoms, but another person may find even mild and infrequent dyskinesia difficult to bear.

A third consideration in designing an individual medication regimen is what kind of activities the person engages in each day. A symptom may have either profound or very little effect on a person's ability to perform an activity, depending on the symptom and on the activity. Someone might continue to pursue an active lifestyle with daily golf or tennis matches in spite of considerable stiffness and slowness, while another person finds the same degree of stiffness and slowness interfering with the use of a computer keyboard in his or her job.

Finally, the timing of symptoms is important, too. For example, a person experiencing particular difficulty getting in and out of bed at night might be helped by a long-acting medication, whereas a person without nighttime problems may do better taking a drug with a shorter duration of action.

People who have Parkinson's disease and their doctors use this type of information—about predominant symptoms, personal reactions to symptoms, lifestyle, and timing of symptoms—in deciding what medication to use and when to use it. These decisions are based on many factors, including how much disability a person experiences, what symptoms need to be relieved, and what side effects need to be avoided so that the person can be comfortable and functional in his or her everyday life and work. As noted earlier, all the currently available medications for Parkinson's disease can only relieve or mask symptoms. They do not prevent the disease's gradual progression. Even if the medication works so effectively that someone reports feeling "back to normal," this does not mean the underlying disease process will no longer progress.

Having said that, we should note that in advanced Parkinson's, medication can protect people from falling and injuring themselves and can certainly delay disability and preserve a person's independent living for many years. There is no urgency about starting medications to relieve mild symptoms, however. Many people who have Parkinson's and their physicians choose to delay the start of medications. Perhaps someone is having mild slowness involving finger dexterity and hand movements on one side but can still function very well, especially if the symptoms only affect their nondominant side. Or a person has a minor tremor in one hand or leg but is not troubled by it. In neither of these instances is there a compelling reason to start drug therapy immediately.

Decisions about medication therapy are often based on the severity of Parkinson's symptoms, but the difference between mild and more advanced symptoms is not always straightforward. Since the symptoms of Parkinson's come on very gradually, people tend to adjust and accommodate to some of the changes over time. For example, it's common for a person who has Parkinson's to describe little to no problems with their daily activities even though they move much slower than normal or their hand has lost most of its agility. There is a fine balance between healthy adjustment to symptoms of a chronic condition and recognizing symptoms that result in substantial disability. Another cause of concern is the impact of Parkinson's symptoms on general fitness and musculoskeletal conditioning. Oftentimes people who have Parkinson's are unaware of the secondary effects that symptoms of slowing and rigidity can have on range of motion and overall level of physical activity. So, decisions about the management of Parkinson's need to take all of these factors into consideration. There is no single "right" way to manage Parkinson's; instead, the best approach is an individualized approach that considers many diverse factors: the patient's history and concerns, the neurological exam, and the overall impact of the symptoms.

IT REMAINS an interesting and open question whether all motor symptoms of Parkinson's disease should be treated early even if causing no discernible impairment in function. There have been outcome studies in early Parkinson's suggesting that if patients' symptoms are treated regardless of whether they are bothersome, as opposed to simply watching and waiting, that six to twelve months later, those patients who were treated early feel better. There isn't evidence that early treatment results in a better outcome years down the road. It seems to be a very individual choice on the part of the patient. If after understanding the diagnosis, the patient finds that the early symptoms are truly not bothersome, there is certainly no harm in delaying treatment, but active follow-up is required with a regular review of how the person is functioning and coping with the symptoms. In this situation, we also strongly encourage patients to participate in clinical research trials designed to evaluate treatments that could slow the progression of the disease. These studies typically need to recruit patients who have little or no disability and can therefore go without the use of "symptomatic" treatment for several months, receiving either a placebo or an active treatment that theoretically could slow progression but should have no impact on improving symptoms.

TAKING ANTIPARKINSON MEDICATIONS

Once the decision is made to take antiparkinson medications, patients should check with their physicians to be sure they are starting
with a low dose. By introducing a medication slowly, we hope the body
will adjust to the drug and the side effects can be minimized. And by
increasing the dose gradually, people who have Parkinson's and their
physicians can determine the optimum dosage that alleviates symptoms yet causes the fewest unwanted side effects (specific side effects
are discussed later in this chapter and in Chapter 13). This means people who have Parkinson's disease must keenly observe how their body
reacts to the drug and tell their doctor what they observe.

Sometimes people take a new drug for one day or even for a single
dose, then discontinue it because it causes adverse effects. This may
be appropriate when the side effect is severe, such as when someone
suddenly develops confusion after starting the new medication. But
given the importance of medications to most people who have Parkinson's, a drug should be given a fair trial before the decision is made that
the individual cannot tolerate it. Several days of taking medication are
generally required for a person to tell whether it is appropriate or not.
Individuals often have an unpleasant initial reaction to a drug, but as it
is continued, their bodies become more tolerant. Also, particularly for
a newly introduced antiparkinson drug, its side effects may not yet be
entirely understood.

If you are concerned about symptoms you suspect are side effects of
antiparkinson drugs, your doctor will be able to tell you whether they
are likely to be related to your medications.

Establishing the relative benefits versus the side effects of a drug
is not easy. Sometimes a person needs to stop taking the drug so the
contrast between how he or she feels with and without the drug is
clearly evident before a final decision is made. Stopping most drugs is
best done by slowly decreasing the dosage over time before discontinuing the drug entirely. Some people will be relieved to be without the
medication; others will discover that the severity of their Parkinson's
symptoms without the drug is unacceptable. This experience may be
delayed with the side effects resolving quickly—that is, the patient

initially feels better, only to experience a significant worsening of Parkinson's symptoms over the next few days. Also, sometimes a person discovers that the "side effects" they were attributing to the new medication continue without the drug; in this case, of course, if the medication was effectively treating Parkinson's symptoms, it can be reintroduced without concern about these specific side effects.

REALISTIC TREATMENT GOALS

The goal of Parkinson's therapy is to preserve people's daily function and comfort. It is unrealistic to expect medications to eliminate every trace of tremor, every trace of slow movement, every trace of gait impairment, or every trace of handwriting difficulty. This doesn't mean such an outcome is impossible; however, to accomplish this with the current medicines, such high doses might be needed that the risk of severe side effects would greatly increase. Most neurologists agree that people should take no more medication than is necessary. As noted above, the tricky part is deciding what is necessary for each individual.

How do we define "preserving people's daily function and comfort"? The definition is fairly elastic—it varies with each person, even among people who have the same symptoms. During an office visit, the neurologist and the patient might conclude, for example, that the patient's daily functioning is not significantly impaired, even though an intermittent resting tremor is present.

You and your doctor will need to balance your medication while considering your ability to function, your physical and emotional comfort, what you and your family desire, and the adverse effects that a medication might have (potential drug interactions as well as long-term complications).

MEDICATION CHANGES

As every person who has Parkinson's disease knows, Parkinson's is a progressive disease. Medications that are effective at one stage of the disorder won't be sufficient later on; importantly, this does not mean that the treatment contributed to a loss of effect with time that would have been avoided by delaying the initiation of treatment. Withholding treatment "until you really need it" does not prevent this problem and often results in living with disability unnecessarily. In addition, increases in dosage may bring side effects. Further, people's dopamine systems gradually become sensitized to levodopa or other medications, and side effects may appear even at the dosage a person has taken for years. Or, because of the combined effects of medications, side effects may appear when a single sleeping pill is added or after surgery or an infection (see Chapter 6).

If you experience any changes in your ability to function or any changes in side effects, be sure to report these to your physician so your medications can be adjusted.

At the higher doses of medication necessary later in the disease, physicians use a risk-benefit analysis to determine the balance between minimizing side effects and alleviating the symptoms as much as possible. There may be a very small difference between the medication regimen that enables a person to function and a regimen that triggers unacceptable side effects. In other words, for a person who has advanced Parkinson's disease, the line between disability and function can be quite thin. Here again, it may be exceedingly useful to seek a consultation with a neurologist who specializes in Parkinson's disease (see Chapter 1).

MEDICATIONS FOR OTHER SYMPTOMS OF PARKINSON'S

In addition to tremor, rigidity, slowness, and gait disorders, Parkinson's produces other symptoms that may require medication. Some 40 percent of people who have Parkinson's, for example, suffer from depression or anxiety. These symptoms often respond to antidepressants and antianxiety agents. Some people who have Parkinson's have muscle spasms in the foot or hand that can be painful. These symptoms generally respond to levodopa or to the dopamine receptor agonists.

As noted in Chapters 4 and 5, some people who have Parkinson's disease have urinary problems. They may need to void more often or feel a sudden, urgent need to void, or they may develop urinary incontinence—the involuntary leakage or spilling of urine. These symptoms can usually be improved by urinary antispasmodic agents; biofeedback training for incontinence can sometimes help, too. For sleep disturbance, sedatives may be prescribed, and laxatives or dietary changes can help with the problem of constipation. Certain drugs may help with bowel motility. (See Chapter 13 for more information on medications for all these symptoms.)

One important thing to remember about these drugs is that they may interact with each other. If some of them have similar side effects, such as drowsiness, their effects when used together may multiply. When a patient starts to take new drugs, we recommend that he or she choose the drug that deals with the most bothersome symptom, beginning with only one drug at a time, at a low dose, and increasing slowly. That way, if a patient has an unacceptable reaction, it will be clear which drug has triggered the reaction.

What is an unacceptable reaction, and what is a tolerable side effect? We address this thorny issue in the remainder of this chapter.

DESIRABLE DRUG EFFECTS AND DRUG SIDE EFFECTS

Although medical research is developing therapies that will reduce the frequency and severity of side effects, we currently do not have medications that eliminate side effects. We do have strategies that can help, however. One hypothesis is that although levodopa is the most potent medication for the symptoms of Parkinson's disease, it may also be the most potent in provoking such side effects as motor fluctuations, dyskinesia, and hallucinations. The dopamine receptor agonists also stimulate the dopamine system in the brain, and COMT inhibitors improve the availability of levodopa to the brain and permit the use of lower levodopa dosages. The use of *combination therapy*—that is, using less levodopa by boosting its effect with other drugs such as dopamine agonists, MAO-B inhibitors, or COMT inhibitors—may result in relief of symptoms with fewer side effects. (See the discussion of levodopa in Chapter 13 for more details.) Lower doses of levodopa combined with medications that enhance its effect may improve symptomatic relief and decrease dopaminergic side effects. However, it should be remembered that levodopa remains the strongest and most potent medication to lessen parkinsonian symptoms.

We should pause here to note again that drug-related side effects and drug-related toxicity are different. A *side effect* is simply an effect that is not the effect for which the drug was designed. Most side effects are undesirable, such as drowsiness when taking an antihistamine or yeast infections that develop during a long course of antibiotics. Some, though, are rather handy. The dry-mouth side effect of anticholinergic medications used for Parkinson's can help control excess saliva or urinary frequency, for example. All medications have the potential to cause side effects, and a physician can rarely predict which patients will have these reactions to medications. These side effects are typically not an indication of a drug allergy, and with the supervision of an expert in Parkinson's diseases, patients should be open to retrying medications that they had quickly abandoned in the past due to a bothersome side effect. For example, stomach upset resulting in vomiting or drop in blood pressure causing fainting with levodopa or dopamine agonists can be very frightening but can often be prevented or successfully managed, allowing the patient to tolerate and benefit from these drugs.

Unlike side effects, *toxicity* from a drug means that the drug causes long-term harm. Levodopa, especially when used for a long time, unquestionably can cause side effects. Based primarily on laboratory experiments, some neuroscientists have asked whether levodopa might also be toxic to neurons in the brain and cause long-term problems. The answer is no: there is no evidence of levodopa toxicity in humans.

The risk of side effects is one of the reasons physicians may choose to delay antiparkinson medication until it is clearly necessary. Some side effects, such as stomach upset, are annoying and can disrupt one's life. But others are more serious. Each of these more serious drug-related symptoms—motor fluctuations, odd dance-like movements called choreiform dyskinesia, and behavioral and psychiatric symptoms—is described below.

If you have drug-related complications, keep in mind that it will take time to manage your symptoms and work out your individual drug regimen. Be sure to tell your doctor if you are having difficulty. The balancing of Parkinson's symptoms and drug-related side effects is often best worked out by a doctor experienced with antiparkinson medications.

Motor Fluctuations

Motor fluctuations are the emergence of periods when Parkinson's symptoms increase because levodopa medication no longer produces the smooth and even effect that is characteristic of the brain's own dopamine-producing system. These motor fluctuations are the most common reason for increasing the amount of each levodopa dose and taking the doses closer together.

We cannot say whether motor fluctuations are caused by levodopa or are a consequence of disease progression. Some researchers believe that if levodopa is taken for a long time, the duration of effect begins to diminish. Others believe that as the disease progresses, the surviving neurons have more and more difficulty both handling and storing the levodopa. It is likely that it is a combination of both disease progression and the effects of levodopa.

Sometimes motor fluctuations are called *on/off fluctuations*. When a person is "on," adequate dopamine is present in the brain and the person can perform tasks almost normally. When a person is "off," insufficient dopamine is present; the person becomes very slow and stiff and has difficulty dressing or walking. The tremor may return and the person may even be unable or barely able to move. Put another way, such overt motor fluctuations occur in advanced Parkinson's disease when the levels of levodopa in the blood and the brain become linked to a person's motor symptoms: if the person weren't taking levodopa, she or he would not have on/off motor fluctuations. However, without levodopa, the person would not experience the "on" benefit but instead would be "off" all the time.

Because people generally do not take Parkinson's medication during the night, in the morning they often experience a period of worsened symptoms until they take their morning dose. People may also experience an "off" period if they forget or delay a dose later in the day. Early in the course of therapy, while Parkinson's symptoms are mild, the medications have a longer duration of effect. Motor fluctuations can be evident even in milder stages of the disease, however; here patients note only a limited increase in symptoms if it's time to take their medications or if they don't take their medications on time. Later, when the symptoms are more advanced, the change from "on" to "off" as the drug's effects wear off becomes more of a problem.

In some people this on/off effect happens at predictable times, such as three hours after taking a levodopa dose (this is called *wearing-off*). But sometimes "off" periods occur at unpredictable times. This, of course, is particularly difficult to handle, because the person doesn't know when it will occur, or where. An individual may be shopping in a store, for example, and suddenly become stiff and frozen, unable to move in the way he or she could move a few minutes earlier.

Caregivers may not understand motor fluctuations. They see a person who has Parkinson's performing in a fairly normal way, and then later in the day asking for help to rise from a chair or walk. A caregiver who does not know about motor fluctuations may think the person is not trying hard enough or is asking to be "babied." Caregivers need to understand about motor fluctuations, and patients need their doctors' help in explaining the problem. The unpredictability of some of the symptoms of Parkinson's can be particularly challenging for caregivers. One needs to find the right balance between doing too much and doing too little to assist the person who has Parkinson's, and this balance may literally change throughout the day based on these fluctuations in medication performance as well as other factors such as fatigue. A healthy relationship built on trust is important; a skilled and compassionate caregiver uses encouragement, reassurance, support, and assistance in different measures to best suit the specific need.

THE PHYSICIAN has the choice of several different approaches for treating motor fluctuations: to increase the total dose of carbidopa/levodopa, to shorten the interval between doses, or to prescribe any number of medications in addition to the levodopa. These additional medications include controlled-release carbidopa/levodopa (Sinemet CR); dopamine receptor agonists such as pramipexole (Mirapex), ropinirole (Requip), and the rotigotine patch; MAO inhibitors such as rasagiline (Azilect); selegiline; apomorphine (Apokyn); and COMT inhibitors such as entacapone (Comtan and Stalevo combined with carbidopa/levodopa) and tolcapone (Tasmar). In some situations, preparing a liquid mixture of carbidopa/levodopa is helpful. Continuous infusions of a levodopa preparation (Duodopa) by a pump directly into the bowel, via a tube placed through the body wall, are used in some Scandinavian and European countries, and this treatment is in clinical research trials in the United States. The doctor may prescribe a diet in which the patient shifts protein intake to the evening (the reasons for this are explained in Chapter 13).

All these methods can be helpful to people who have Parkinson's who develop motor fluctuations. Because some of these drugs to control motor fluctuations have their *own* side effects, if you are taking drugs of this type you will need to work closely with your doctor to find the combination that works for you.

Involuntary Movements

Dyskinesia (from *dys,* meaning "not correct" or "difficult," and *kinesia,* referring to movement) is a condition in which a person makes generally odd, writhing, random, wiggly movements. Because the movements can be dance-like, this is called *choreiform dyskinesia* (from the Greek *chorea,* meaning "dance"). They may involve the face, mouth, tongue, head, arms, trunk, or legs. They can vary from just the fingers moving around a bit to whole body movements, with the entire trunk wiggling and twisting around so much that it becomes difficult to walk. These irregular movements are not like Parkinson's regular, rhythmical tremor.

Before medications were available to treat the stiffness, slowness, and walking problems of Parkinson's disease, people who had Parkinson's didn't have dyskinetic movements. Parkinson's medications are an effort to replace parts of a biochemical system that is not functioning properly in the brain, and sometimes they have odd effects. The brain's system may become sensitive to the Parkinson's medications over time, resulting in these dance-like movements. Movement control consists of a highly complex and intricate group of systems and, when damaged, is difficult to repair.

Dyskinesia occurs in a number of temporal patterns. The most common time sequence is onset of dyskinesia at the peak effect of the medications (*peak-dose dyskinesia*). In other people, dyskinesia occurs both when the effects of the medication are starting (beginning of dose) and when the effects are waning (end of dose). This combination is referred to as *diphasic dyskinesia* or the *dyskinesia-improvement-dyskinesia* (DID) *pattern.* Involuntary dyskinesia can also take the form of postures and often-painful muscle spasms known as *dystonia* (*tonia* refers to the tone of the muscles). Dystonia occurs most often when drug levels are very low, but may also occur in association with the dance-like movements known as *choreodystonic dyskinesia.*

Levodopa-induced peak-dose dyskinesia eventually develops in most patients who obtain a good response to levodopa (i.e., in some respects they can be seen as a "necessary evil"), and they are often an indication that the medication is indeed resulting in benefit. They can always be reversed by reducing the amount of antiparkinson medications the patient is receiving. If the patient is taking only carbidopa/levodopa (Sinemet), reducing the dosage will reduce the movements. If a patient is taking carbidopa/levodopa along with dopamine receptor agonists, COMT, or MAO-B inhibitors, a reduction in one or more of these other medications will also reduce the frequency and severity of the dyskinesia.

If the dosage of the antiparkinson medication is reduced in order to improve the abnormal movements, almost invariably the resting tremor, gait difficulty, or slowness of movement will worsen. Many patients are not aware that they are demonstrating dyskinesias and most will admit that the abnormal movements are not as concerning as they had anticipated when they began treatment. Given a choice, many people prefer the times when they experience peak-dose dyskinesia to the times when they are "off" and suffer from increased slowness, rigidity, and tremor. Experienced neurologists use a number of strategies to find the proper balance of these medications. Some people who have Parkinson's are overly concerned about the possibility of developing dyskinesia, to the point that they resist beginning levodopa therapy even when their symptoms are causing profound impairment in their daily activities and quality of life. We strongly advise against this misguided delay in using what is currently the most effective treatment for Parkinson's disease.

Behavioral and Psychiatric Side Effects

A number of antiparkinson drugs, including levodopa and the dopamine agonists, may cause behavioral changes or psychiatric side effects. At some point, almost half of people who have Parkinson's will have some of these effects. They range from vivid dreams, nightmares, and nonthreatening visual hallucinations to delusional states, paranoia, agitation, disorientation, and psychosis. (These symptoms are also discussed in Chapter 6.)

These drug-related effects can be reduced and often abolished by lowering the dose of levodopa or other antiparkinson medications. As noted before, the challenge is to diminish side effects without allowing Parkinson's symptoms to become unacceptably severe.

Sometimes the behavioral disorders gradually progress, beginning with vivid dreams, moving on to benign hallucinations, and ending with psychosis. But some people experience vivid dreams and never develop hallucinations or delusions. And others suddenly develop paranoia and psychosis with little or no warning.

Drug-induced hallucinations and delusions usually occur in the person who has advanced Parkinson's who is taking several drugs, including dopamine receptor agonists, COMT inhibitors, MAO inhibitors, amantadine, and anticholinergics. Behavioral abnormalities are certainly possible when carbidopa/levodopa or any other antiparkinson drug is administered alone, but they also occur as combined effects of many antiparkinson medications.

As discussed in Chapter 6, perhaps most of these symptoms are better thought of as resulting from excessive dopamine stimulation within the brain possibly resulting from a variety of antiparkinson medications, either alone or in combination. Sometimes an underlying illness such as a pneumonia or a bladder infection (even a very mild one with minimal symptoms) can trigger psychiatric symptoms. There is some medical disagreement about whether the hallucinations and delusions really are side effects or are signs of the progression of Parkinson's disease. The evidence points to the drugs, but the underlying disease clearly serves as a predisposition.

Vivid Dreams and Nighttime Vocalizations. People who take dopaminergic medication frequently report vivid dreams and nightmares, which appear to be an intensification of normal dreaming. Many people explain that, formerly, they were not accustomed to dreaming or to remembering their dreams. Now, not only do they remember their dreams, but the dreams have a lifelike, vivid quality with clearer definition of themes and figures.

The dreamers often talk, call out, or thrash about in bed. They don't remember such activities, but their bed partners often comment on this nighttime behavior. Sometimes this activity in sleep is so vigorous or violent that the bed partner may have to move to another bed or another room to sleep. This loud and vigorous nighttime behavior sometimes is a manifestation of REM (rapid eye movement) sleep behavior disorder (RBD). The doctor may suggest an overnight sleep recording in a sleep laboratory to better understand why a person is behaving so strangely while asleep.

Hallucinations. Antiparkinson therapy may also cause nonthreatening "benign" visual hallucinations. At first the visual hallucinations are often startling to the patient, but he or she quickly adapts to their presence. Oddly enough, many people become accustomed to these visual hallucinations and are not alarmed by them. It is common for a doctor to ask whether the patient is experiencing hallucinations such as seeing people, animals, or insects that shouldn't be there, and, much to the astonishment of the family, the person responds, "Oh, yes, I see people in my house" or "An object like a rolled-up sweater often looks like an animal to me." In many cases, people understand the visual hallucinations are not real, and they commonly note, "Yes, I still have my nighttime visitors, but I know they aren't real" or "Yes, there is still a dog in my living room, but he doesn't bother me."

Generally, it is when people start having difficulty discriminating the visual hallucinations from real events that serious problems begin. Family members may be surprised as the behavior of the person who has Parkinson's becomes increasingly unpredictable: he or she may call the emergency number (911) to report prowlers, for example, or set out food for the visual apparitions, or turn up the air conditioning in order to accommodate the visitors. One husband, whose wife saw many small children in the house, reported, "I don't find it so hard to live with the hallucinations but I do object to having to clean up all the milk and cookies that she constantly puts out for them."

Delusions. People on long-term levodopa therapy may also become paranoid. Common paranoid themes such as believing someone is stealing their money or believing their spouse is having an affair may cause serious disruption within the family. Psychosis is a serious mental disorder in which an individual is unable to distinguish the delusions from reality. Both paranoia and psychosis require prompt medical intervention.

When drug-induced psychosis is severe, the patient may be severely disoriented, unable to discriminate what is real from what is not. Hospitalization is essential for the safety of the patient. In the hospital, a new medication regimen can be started. Again, simultaneously controlling Parkinson's symptoms and side effects takes much expertise and, often, repeated efforts.

IF YOU ARE TAKING MEDICATIONS for Parkinson's, be sure you understand the issues surrounding these drugs and talk to your doctor about all the ins and outs. Some of the medication decisions are not easy, and you and your doctor will have to decide what is best for you.

CHAPTER 13

Drug Therapies

- *Why are there so many different kinds of medications to treat the symptoms of Parkinson's disease?*
- *Which drug combinations are most effective?*
- *What are the options if a drug has unacceptable side effects?*

Drugs are very important in the treatment of Parkinson's so that people who have this disease can continue to function well in their lives. In this chapter we describe the primary drugs used for Parkinson's, beginning with the most commonly used (Table 13.1). As we consider these medications, it is important to keep in mind that the motor control system of the brain is enormously complex and adding drugs to the system affected by Parkinson's disease can only approximate the way this system normally works. Nonetheless, these drugs represent a significant improvement over what was available even ten years ago.

LEVODOPA

Levodopa, first used in the 1960s, continues to be the single most dramatic development in the treatment of people who have Parkinson's disease (see Chapter 11). The drug revolutionized Parkinson's therapy, suddenly allowing people who had been wheelchair-bound and having extraordinary difficulty performing the activities of daily living to regain much of their ability to function more normally. There was even a short-lived hope that levodopa might be a cure for Parkinson's disease.

TABLE 13.1
PRIMARY DRUGS USED TO RELIEVE SYMPTOMS OF PARKINSON'S DISEASE

Drugs for motor symptoms
Levodopa
Levodopa plus peripheral dopa decarboxylase inhibitors (Ddis)
Dopamine receptor agonists
Levodopa plus COMT inhibitors (catechol-O-methyltransferase
  inhibitors)
MAO inhibitors (monoamine oxidase inhibitors)
Anticholinergics
Amantadine

Drugs for other symptoms
Tricyclic antidepressants
Selective serotonin reuptake inhibitors (SSRIs)
Cholinesterase inhibitors
Benzodiazepines
Sedatives
Atypical antipsychotic agents
Stool softeners
Fiber-rich preparations

Within a year or two of the drug's introduction, however, it became clear that levodopa provided dramatic symptomatic relief even as the underlying disease continued to progress.

As described in Chapter 11, a problem with levodopa therapy, which became clear soon after the drug was introduced, is that the body converts levodopa to dopamine in the bloodstream, which not only prevents levodopa from reaching the brain (where it is needed) but also causes severe nausea and vomiting. To solve the gastrointestinal problems and allow levodopa to reach the brain intact, treatment was developed that combines levodopa with a *peripheral dopa decarboxylase inhibitor* (DDI), which blocks the body's natural conversion of levodopa to dopamine in the bloodstream. Because DDIs cannot cross the blood-brain barrier, once levodopa reaches the brain, it can enter the brain to be converted to dopamine unaffected by the DDI, which is left behind in the bloodstream. Levodopa can be taken alone, but because so many people develop nausea and vomiting when taking levodopa alone, it is seldom prescribed this way. When we say "levodopa therapy," we mean a combination of levodopa and a DDI.

Another limitation of levodopa therapy is that the dopamine-producing nerve cells in the substantia nigra, as they are increasingly affected by the disease over time, become less able to convert levodopa to dopamine. To stimulate the dopamine receptors, then, many people who have moderate or advanced Parkinson's disease take a *dopamine receptor agonist* along with a DDI/levodopa medication. The dopamine receptor agonist mimics the activity of dopamine at the dopamine receptor, stimulates the transmission of nerve signals, and smooths out the symptoms of Parkinson's (see Chapter 11).

We should pause to note again that levodopa is also useful for diagnosing Parkinson's disease. If a person begins taking levodopa and experiences a dramatic improvement in symptoms, this improvement is helpful in confirming the clinical diagnosis of Parkinson's, although people who have other parkinsonian disorders also may obtain substantial benefit, at least initially. When a person who has parkinsonian symptoms does not notice that his or her symptoms respond to levodopa, the correct diagnosis is likely to be a type of parkinsonism other than Parkinson's disease. On the other hand, we do not recommend the levodopa challenge using a single dose of levodopa in untreated patients to make a diagnosis. The initial response is often an unreliable predictor of later response, and we have seen patients incorrectly told that they did not have Parkinson's disease on the basis of a negative test. Later in treatment there are times when the patient and physician are unsure whether or not the symptoms are responding to levodopa. In this situation, the medication may need to be gradually withdrawn and perhaps later reintroduced, with reexamination of the patient when not taking and when taking the medication.

DDIs

Carbidopa and *benserazide* are the two DDIs commonly used today. The combination of levodopa and carbidopa is known by the trade name Sinemet (*Sine Emesis*—that is, without vomiting), and the combination of levodopa and benserazide is known as Prolopa or Madopar. Sinemet is marketed in the United States and most other countries

TABLE 13.2
CARBIDOPA/LEVODOPA PREPARATIONS

Generic Name	Trademark Name
Carbidopa/levodopa (10/100, 25/100, 25/250)	Sinemet (10/100, 25/100, 25/250)
Carbidopa/levodopa CR (25/100, 50/200)	Sinemet CR (25/100, 50/200)
Carbidopa/levodopa ODT (10/100, 25/100, 25/250)	Parcopa
Benserazide/levodopa	Madopar, Prolopa (12.5/50, 25/100, 50/200) Madopar HBS

throughout the world, and Prolopa (or Madopar) is marketed in Canada and many European countries. There is very little difference in the pharmacologic properties of the two DDIs.

Many different formulations of levodopa and DDIs are sold today (Table 13.2). Carbidopa/levodopa is available as a generic preparation. The dose of the two drugs in the preparation is designated as a fraction: the numerator is the amount of carbidopa in each tablet, and the denominator the amount of levodopa. For example, a combination of 10/100 is composed of 10 milligrams of carbidopa and 100 milligrams of levodopa. Carbidopa/levodopa is available in combination pills of 10/100, 25/100, and 25/250. In Canada and some European countries the convention is to give the levodopa dose as the numerator and the DDI dose as the denominator (in other words, the levodopa/DDI ratio). Thus, Prolopa (or Madopar) is available in the following combinations: 50/12.5, 100/25, and 200/50 (or 12.5/50, 25/100, and 50/200 using the U.S. convention, as in Table 13.2).

Typically, the larger the amount of DDI given the better, especially early in the use of levodopa, when doses of carbidopa may be so low that they are not adequate to inhibit the enzyme activity in the body so as to facilitate passage of levodopa into the brain. Most patients require a minimum of 75 to 150 milligrams of carbidopa or benserazide each day. At the one-to-four (1:4) carbidopa/levodopa ratio (25/100 tablets), the patient usually starts with one 25/100 tablet three times each day. Tablets with a carbidopa/levodopa ratio of 1:10 (25/250 tablets) are used for some patients, but there is little difference between the 1:10 and 1:4 ratios in practical terms. The 1:4 ratio may be more useful for someone who has gastrointestinal side effects from therapy.

For some people, nausea and vomiting are a significant problem, particularly if this side effect limits the amount of carbidopa/levodopa they can take. When even the 1:4 ratio does not supply enough carbidopa, the person may benefit from an additional dose of carbidopa alone, called Lodosyn.

Carbidopa/levodopa is also sold in a *controlled-release* formulation known as Sinemet CR, available in doses of 25/100 or 50/200. The controlled-release formulations of Sinemet provide a slower release of levodopa into the bloodstream, which produces a somewhat longer duration of action. There was some speculation that Sinemet CR might produce fewer long-term side effects than immediate-release Sinemet. However, a five-year study comparing Sinemet to Sinemet CR in people who have early Parkinson's disease did not reveal any significant difference in the frequency or severity of levodopa-related side effects.

Some Parkinson's symptoms crop up just as the levodopa is wearing off, and Sinemet CR's controlled release can help smooth them out. These symptoms include motor fluctuations, end-of-dose wearing-off fluctuations or on/off fluctuations (people become suddenly stiff and frozen when the medication wears off), and nighttime immobility and sleep disruption. In the early morning, when drug levels are low, some people have difficulties with increased slowness, stiffness, or foot cramps. When these fluctuations are frequent or unpredictable, Sinemet CR may contribute to the problem by taking longer to "kick in" and being less reliably absorbed. In this case, the persons may have a more reliable, albeit still fluctuating, response with the standard levodopa formulations.

Carbidopa/levodopa is also available as an orally dispersible tablet (ODT) that can conveniently be placed in the mouth to dissolve. Carbidopa/levodopa can also be administered as a homemade liquid preparation, which is particularly effective for people who are having a lot of trouble with on/off fluctuations. The advantage is that, in this form, the drug is quickly and easily absorbed from the digestive tract; the disadvantage is that people must take the liquid preparation about every hour. As mentioned in Chapter 12, a special formulation of levodopa

(Levodopa-Carbidopa Intestinal Gel [LCIG], or Duodopa) given by a pump through the body wall directly into the small intestine is available in some Scandinavian and European countries, and this will eventually be marketed in North America.

Drugs often act in different ways, depending on whether they are taken with food or not. Levodopa is no exception. It is best absorbed through the digestive tract on an empty stomach, so the optimum time to take it is twenty to thirty minutes before a meal or two hours after a meal. If the levodopa is causing nausea or gastrointestinal discomfort, it should be taken at mealtime or soon after meals. However, because levodopa taken with food is not absorbed as well as levodopa taken on an empty stomach, someone who takes levodopa at mealtime may not get as much effective medication and therefore as much symptom improvement as he or she would otherwise. Patients are often incorrectly advised by their pharmacies that they need to take levodopa with meals. Again, this is only necessary if nausea occurs when the medication is taken without food. Taking it with food should be avoided if food is having a deleterious effect on drug absorption and motor fluctuations are aggravated. The effectiveness of the time-release formulation, Sinemet CR, is less affected by meals, and this may be a distinct advantage. However, as mentioned above, Sinemet CR is somewhat less reliably absorbed, and this can cause problems in the later stage of treatment—taking longer to give any benefit, and some doses not working as reliably as others.

When Should Treatment Start?

There is controversy about when a person who has Parkinson's disease should start levodopa treatment. This is a difficult question. We don't yet know whether starting levodopa early increases the risk of chronic complications of levodopa therapy (such as motor fluctuations, dyskinesia, hallucinations, and delusions) or whether these complications occur simply because the disease is becoming more severe—in which case the length of time a person has been taking levodopa is not an issue. In recent clinical trials comparing early use of levodopa with early use of dopamine agonists, early levodopa treatment led to better motor performance but more motor fluctuations and dyskinesia.

Early use of dopamine agonists resulted in less dyskinesia and fewer motor fluctuations, as well as significant improvement in motor performance, but the latter effect was not as great as with levodopa treatment. However, the overall outcomes after ten years, when all patients are generally on levodopa with other drugs, are probably no different. We discuss this further in the next chapter.

In general, though, doctors agree that people should start taking levodopa when their Parkinson's symptoms begin to interfere significantly with their daily functioning and quality of life. As discussed in Chapter 12, this varies from person to person. One person may begin to use levodopa when he or she has difficulty using a computer keyboard at work or when handwriting has deteriorated so much that it's no longer legible to others. Someone else may decide to start levodopa therapy when he or she can no longer prepare meals for the family or enjoy recreational activities such as golf or tennis. Starting treatment with levodopa markedly improves the symptoms of Parkinson's for the vast majority of people.

People who have Parkinson's can start with either the original, immediate-release Sinemet (carbidopa/levodopa) or Sinemet CR (the controlled-release formulation). The immediate-release preparation takes effect earlier and the effect may be more evident—after taking it for a time, people often feel it "kick in"—but its action does not last as long as that of the controlled-release drug. With the controlled-release form, people can wait somewhat longer between doses, but the beneficial effects are more subtle.

Some people worry about starting levodopa "too early" in the disease, and many of our patients ask whether the beneficial effects of levodopa become weaker after many years of use. The fact is that levodopa remains effective for Parkinson's symptoms for the duration of the illness. But the disease does progress and the symptoms do become more severe. Although levodopa continues to relieve and improve symptoms, the extent to which it can restore function becomes less satisfactory with time. In other words, levodopa does not lose its potency over time and people do not develop tolerance to it, but the underlying Parkinson's symptoms progress so that the improvement is not as complete as it once was.

Also, the way in which people react to levodopa changes slightly as symptoms worsen. Initially, people who have Parkinson's have a smooth response to carbidopa/levodopa—that is, they take two to three doses of medication and the effects last all day. Later in the disease they begin to notice when the drug wears off, and they begin to develop end-of-dose wearing-off fluctuations or on/off fluctuations. Then the dose and frequency of the drug generally need to be increased.

People who have early Parkinson's have more and more alternatives to levodopa for symptomatic relief, including dopamine agonists and the MAO inhibitors rasagiline, selegiline, and increasing numbers may begin to use levodopa somewhat later in the course of their illness. Whether the use of these alternatives to levodopa for symptomatic relief is better in the long term remains unclear.

The Protein Redistribution Diet

As discussed in Chapter 12, levodopa, even with DDIs, can be associated with disruptive side effects such as motor fluctuations. These motor fluctuations occur in somewhat more advanced Parkinson's, when relief of symptoms becomes dependent upon a narrower range of levodopa levels in the brain. Consequently, when the amount of dopamine in the brain becomes too low, people's tremor, stiffness, slowness, and walking problems reappear. If people notice they have motor fluctuations when they eat a meal containing protein (meat, cheese, dairy products, or beans), they may benefit from the protein redistribution diet. This diet reduces the intake of protein during the daytime hours without reducing overall protein consumption. All it does is shift protein intake from breakfast and lunch to the evening meal.

Levodopa, like the building blocks from which proteins are made, is an amino acid. The proteins we eat are largely broken down into their amino acids in our digestive system, which does not discriminate between levodopa and the amino acids from food protein. As the food amino acids compete with the levodopa for passage through the wall of the small intestine into the bloodstream, the levodopa may have difficulty being properly absorbed into the blood. In fact, some of the levodopa does not enter the bloodstream but instead is sluiced down the digestive tract and out of the body.

There is probably a second whammy in this scenario. The amino acids derived from food probably also compete with the levodopa for passage from the bloodstream into the brain. To a certain extent, these amino acids can block levodopa from getting into the brain.

Some people, generally those with more advanced Parkinson's symptoms, report that when they take Sinemet (carbidopa/levodopa) and have a high-protein meal such as a hamburger, the dose of Sinemet does not "kick in" and take effect. These individuals may notice improvement in their symptoms if they limit protein during the day, shifting their major protein intake to dinnertime (which, however, may mean that the response to levodopa in the evening could be compromised).

The protein redistribution diet is *not* meant to reduce the total amount of protein in the diet—that would have serious consequences for a person's general health. Instead, the diet is designed to shift the protein intake to later in the day, so levodopa absorption is enhanced during the earlier hours and daytime motor function is improved.

If you are taking carbidopa/levodopa and have *not* noticed any adverse effects from dietary protein, you are unlikely to notice any benefit from following the protein redistribution diet. Generally, only people who have experienced obvious end-of-dose wearing-off or on/off fluctuations will notice a beneficial effect of protein redistribution. And even then, only a small proportion of such people are likely to benefit.

Special diets are available that deliver calories with a specific carbohydrate/protein ratio in an attempt to minimize the disruption that protein may cause for some people who have Parkinson's. These diets can be obtained from Parkinson's disease organizations. We recommend that, before using these diets, you establish that you really need to make this dietary change and discuss the protein redistribution diet with a physician experienced in treating Parkinson's disease.

People who have early Parkinson's who are not taking any medications have no reason to follow the protein redistribution diet. Nor should people who are taking only selegiline, rasagiline, dopamine agonists, anticholinergics, or amantadine use the diet—these drugs do not compete with dietary protein.

In summary, then, people who are taking carbidopa/levodopa, who find their motor symptoms are relieved by this therapy, and who do not have motor fluctuations or levodopa dosage failures will not benefit from a protein redistribution diet. The diet should be used only by people who report a clear loss of carbidopa/levodopa effect when they take the drug in conjunction with a protein meal, and by people who are experiencing poorly controlled motor fluctuations.

Drugs That Enhance Levodopa and Dopamine

The conversion of levodopa to dopamine within the brain involves the dopamine-producing neurons that are located in the substantia nigra and communicate with the striatum (caudate and putamen), to which they deliver their dopamine. These are the very neurons affected by the disease process in Parkinson's (Figure 13.1). Therefore, it is not surprising that as the disease increasingly affects these neurons over time, there are fewer neurons to handle the metabolic conversion of levodopa to dopamine. Other cells probably take over this conversion, but these cells simply release the dopamine immediately, without the normal control or storage exercised by normally functioning dopaminergic neurons.

One way around this problem has been the development of drugs that *mimic dopamine* in directly stimulating dopamine receptors (the dopamine receptor agonists) and drugs that *inhibit the breakdown of dopamine* in the body and thus increase the levels available to the brain (the COMT and MAO inhibitors).

Dopamine Agonists

When dopamine is released by the axon of a neuron, it passes across an extremely small space (the synaptic cleft) and excites dopamine receptors in an adjacent neuron. As a dopamine receptor is activated, information (the signal) is passed to this next neuron in the pathway, and then is passed along to the next neuron in a similar fashion.

A *dopamine receptor agonist* is a drug that mimics the activity of dopamine at the dopamine receptor. It does not have to be metabolized (converted to another substance) within the brain to become active. The potential advantages of such a drug include the alleviation

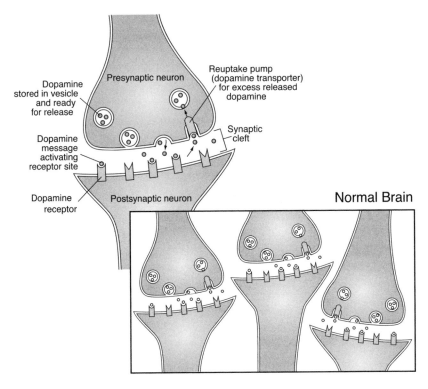

Dopamine stored in vesicle and ready for release

Presynaptic neuron

Reuptake pump (dopamine transporter) for excess released dopamine

Dopamine message activating receptor site

Synaptic cleft

Dopamine receptor

Postsynaptic neuron

Normal Brain

Parkinson's Brain

Dopamine receptor agonist

FIGURE 13.1 In the topmost illustration a normal synapse is depicted with the presynaptic and postsynaptic neuron. Shown here is the cellular machinery, which includes dopamine stored in vesicles and dopamine released into the synapse, where it acts on the dopamine receptors to communicate with the postsynaptic neuron. In the panel depicting the normal brain, normal presynaptic and postsynaptic neurons are present, and therefore motor commands and motor activities can be carried out normally. In the panel depicting the Parkinson's brain, the number of presynaptic dopamine neurons that originate in the substantia nigra is reduced. This leaves fewer dopamine neurons in the substantia nigra to communicate dopamine-related messages, and therefore the symptoms of Parkinson's disease emerge.

of Parkinson's symptoms and the possibility of a smoother effect, since the drug doesn't have to be metabolized by the very neurons that are affected by the disease process.

In the early 1970s, the first dopamine receptor agonist, *bromocriptine* (Parlodel), proved effective in treating the basic symptoms of Parkinson's disease. For well over ten years, bromocriptine was the only dopamine receptor agonist available to treat Parkinson's. Then, in the 1980s, *pergolide* (Permax) was introduced. And in 1997 two new dopamine receptor agonists, *pramipexole* (Mirapex) and *ropinirole* (Requip) were approved by the U.S. Food and Drug Administration (FDA) for the treatment of both early and advanced Parkinson's disease. These four dopamine receptor agonists work using the same general mechanism, but they are not all the same. Dopamine agonists not widely available include *lisuride* and *cabergoline. Apomorphine* is an injectable form of dopamine agonist that we discuss later in this chapter. *Rotigitine* (Neupro), a dopamine agonist delivered via skin patch, was initially approved by the FDA but then withdrawn from the market because of crystallization problems of the drug within the patch. This problem has been corrected and FDA approval is granted and Neupro is back on the market and is available.

As noted in Chapter 11, there are at least five types of dopamine receptors in the brain, called D_1, D_2, D_3, D_4, and D_5. Each dopamine receptor agonist has a slightly different profile of how it acts on these five different receptors; however, it is still not clear whether or how this affects their overall benefit and side effect profile. All dopamine receptor agonists must stimulate the D_2 receptor in order to relieve the major symptoms of Parkinson's disease. For example, pergolide stimulates the D_1 and D_2 receptors; pramipexole and ropinirole stimulate D_2 and D_3 receptors. There is mounting evidence that the D_3 receptor is involved more in aspects of personality and emotion than in motor control. For example, stimulation of D_3 may affect symptoms of depression, apathy, and passivity.

Each of the agonists can be combined with carbidopa/levodopa, and this combination is often useful in moderate or advanced Parkinson's. Some physicians prescribe a dopamine agonist alone as the initial drug in early Parkinson's disease (called *monotherapy*), delaying the introduction of levodopa. Some physicians attempt to reduce the total amount of levodopa to which the person is exposed over the years. Most commonly, though, people start using the agonists after they have been taking carbidopa/levodopa for a number of years and are beginning to experience some of the long-term problems associated with this medication, such as motor fluctuations or dyskinesia. All of the agonists have proved effective in increasing the amount of "on" time, when the person is experiencing a beneficial antiparkinson effect. Agonists also reduce the time spent feeling slow and stiff and thereby improve overall functioning.

All agonists can produce the side effects lethargy, dizziness, low blood pressure, swollen ankles, and psychiatric disturbances. The agonist must be started at a very low dosage, and the dosage must then be titrated up very slowly (titrate means to observe or measure any change in effect with each small increase in dose). The slow, gradual introduction may avoid such side effects as dizziness and nausea. Because several agonists are available, if the first one is not effective or causes too many side effects, a different agonist can be taken. People who can't tolerate one may do very well with another. Dopamine agonists also need to be withdrawn very slowly to avoid a dopamine agonist withdrawal syndrome, characterized by irritability, depression, and fatigue.

Another possibility to avoid side effects is to use a dopamine receptor blocker called domperidone. Dopamine circulating in the bloodstream in large amounts can stimulate the brain's vomiting center, because this center uses an outside-the-brain blood supply. Dopamine agonists cause nausea by directly affecting the vomiting center in the same way. Domperidone blocks the dopamine receptors in the body but not those in the brain and thus can prevent the dopamine agonists from stimulating the vomiting center, but it does not interfere with the agonists' effectiveness for Parkinson's symptoms. Domperidone is available in Canada, Europe, and Israel but not in the United States. People in the United States who need domperidone can obtain it for their personal use by asking their neurologists for a prescription, then arranging for the prescription to be filled outside the country.

Agonists can also cause the side effects of dyskinesia and psychiatric problems, which are associated with the total amount of stimulation the dopamine system is receiving. As we have seen, levodopa stimulates the dopamine system, and by using a slightly different method, so do the agonists. As a result, when an agonist is added to the medications, hallucinations or dyskinesia may either worsen or emerge for the first time. If dyskinesia becomes troublesome, the levodopa dosage must be reduced gradually as the dopamine agonist is introduced. A common error is to conclude that a person cannot tolerate the dopamine agonists when the real difficulty is that levodopa needs to be reduced. On the other hand, if hallucinations develop while introducing a dopamine agonist, the agonist needs to be reduced. Psychiatric side effects are more likely with the agonists.

Another mistake is to simply stop the carbidopa/levodopa and introduce the dopamine agonist. This almost always results in an unacceptable worsening of the Parkinson's symptoms. In this situation, people often mistakenly believe that the agonist is making their symptoms worse.

People who have Parkinson's need to know that the effect of an agonist feels different from the effect of levodopa. Sometimes people decide that an agonist is not helping because the treatment does not "kick in" and give them the sudden burst of motor energy that accompanies the transition from "off" to "on" with levodopa. Agonists do not "kick in." They work more slowly to improve motor performance and their effect also wears off more gradually, so they don't produce the more dramatic changes that people may observe with levodopa.

Many people who have Parkinson's and their physicians give up on dopamine receptor agonists too quickly if no benefit is obtained early in the course of therapy with a low dose. And many patients fail to obtain the benefits of agonists because the drug is simply not introduced properly. Generally, a persistent effort to get to higher doses results in considerable benefit.

New Developments in the Use of Agonists. Another controversy in the treatment of Parkinson's is about how agonists are used, which grew partly out of the original hopes for these medications. Because the long-term use of levodopa often produces drug-related side effects, physicians hoped that the agonists would be "levodopa-sparing agents"—in other words, that the agonists could be used for a while, postponing the need for levodopa until later in the disease.

Initially, bromocriptine was used alone in just such a way, but the large doses required caused disruptive side effects including lethargy, dizziness, low blood pressure, and psychiatric disturbances. All the agonists produce similar side effects, but, as already mentioned, people who have side effects with one agonist may very well tolerate another.

Pramipexole, ropinirole, and rotigotine have been found to work as monotherapies (used alone, without levodopa) in early Parkinson's. They have been effective in reducing symptoms including tremor, rigidity, and slowness, and many researchers have been favorably impressed that people generally tolerate these drugs well. Pergolide has also proved an effective monotherapy in early Parkinson's. Unfortunately, reports indicate that pergolide is associated with cardiac valve abnormalities. A number of patients taking pergolide were found to have scarred cardiac valves and the drug was removed from the market. (Cabergoline, which is not marketed for Parkinson's disease in North America, also seems to be associated with this risk.) The newer agonists, pramipexole, ropinirole, and rotigotine have not been associated with this problem.

Nonetheless, the most common use of dopamine agonists is in combination with levodopa in order to maximize relief of Parkinson's symptoms. The hope once again is that using the agonists in early Parkinson's will cut down on the side effects associated with antiparkinson drugs later in the course of the illness.

Studies comparing the use of the agonists ropinirole, pramipexole, and pergolide versus carbidopa/levodopa as monotherapy in patients with early Parkinson's have been conducted. The studies demonstrate that early use of agonists decreases the frequency of dyskinesia. However, in these studies levodopa use resulted in more improvement in the motor disability of Parkinson's and a better quality of life as measured by special tests. The question now is whether the reduction in dyskinesia and motor fluctuations in the early years is of long-term significance in the management of Parkinson's disease. There is no compelling evidence that prevention of early, mild dyskinesias is of long-term significance in the management of Parkinson's, since all patients eventually require levodopa, and, if motor fluctuations and dyskinesias are going to develop, then initiating treatment with a dopamine agonist probably only postpones these symptoms in the early years when they are not that bothersome. In fact, overall, the use of dopamine agonists compared to levodopa results in increased side effects including ankle swelling, livedo reticularis (mild rash and swelling on the ankles), impulse control disorders and other behavioral problems, postural hypotension (low blood pressure on standing), and increased economic costs. Dopamine agonists remain very useful in combination with levodopa to treat tremor, slowness and stiffness, motor fluctuations, and dyskinesias in Parkinson's.

Which Agonist Is Best? There have been almost no studies directly comparing the different agonists. In general, they all help. We have a great deal of information about how each one works, and research is providing more information all the time. What we don't know is how any individual will react to each of the different agonists.

If you are planning to take a dopamine receptor agonist, your doctor will need to make what appears to be the best choice for you; then you will need to monitor your body to see how well your symptoms respond to the agonist, what the side effects are, and how you feel about the changes. If one agonist doesn't work, try another. Your doctor will also have to make a recommendation about whether you take a dopamine receptor agonist or levodopa as your first medication and whether you take it as a combination drug for moderate or advanced Parkinson's.

Keep in mind that agonists are often underprescribed and that they may be beneficial for you. Many physicians are reluctant to prescribe adequate dosages of these medications, and it takes time to carefully and slowly titrate the dosage up into the range where the agonists become effective; given the nature of the formulations and effective dosages, this is especially the case with ropinirole more than with pramipexole. This requires patience on the part of both the patient and the physician, especially while dealing with the various side effects. In the long run, however, it is often worthwhile tolerating side effects in exchange for major motor benefits. Both ropinirole and pramipexole are now available in long-acting forms, which provide an easier route method of administration for patients. Of course, the longer-acting form is more expensive. The skin patch method of administering rotigotine, applied once per day, is also very convenient. On the other hand, skin reactions to the patch are unique to this formulation and these can sometimes be quite bothersome and occasionally force discontinuation of the drug.

Apomorphine (Apokyn) is an injectable dopamine agonist marketed in the United States. Apomorphine has the same beneficial effect and the same side effects as the other dopamine agonists we have just discussed. It is the only agonist that is self-administered by subcutaneous (just under the skin) injection. It is used most often in conjunction with carbidopa/levodopa and orally administered dopamine agonists to cut short an "off" period. Some people who have Parkinson's notice that an "off" period may last sixty to ninety minutes, despite taking their next scheduled medication. An apomorphine injection often turns a person back "on" within ten to twenty minutes.

Initiating therapy with apomorphine is not just a simple matter of a new prescription and instructions. If you and your doctor decide you should begin this therapy, the drug and injection equipment must be ordered in advance from a special pharmacy. Then, three days before your appointment with the doctor to start therapy, you must begin to take trimethobenzamide (Tigan), a medication to prevent the nausea that apomorphine might cause. On the day of your appointment, you do not take your morning antiparkinson medication, and you arrive at your appointment in an "off" state. You and your family receive instructions on how to use the injection, and then the medical staff will determine the apomorphine dose that is correct for you in a stepwise manner. The whole procedure may take one to three hours. In addition to being used for this intermittent "rescue" therapy, in some countries apomorphine is given by continuous infusion with special pumps.

COMT Inhibitors and MAO Inhibitors

The COMT (catechol-O-methyltransferase) inhibitors and MAO-B (monoamine oxidase type B) inhibitors operate on enzyme systems to increase the amount of dopamine available to the brain's motor control system. As we described in Chapter 11 and earlier in this chapter, when someone takes a tablet of carbidopa/levodopa, some of the levodopa is hijacked by enzymes and is changed to dopamine in the bloodstream;

this dopamine cannot get into the brain to be used by the motor control system.

One of the enzymes that hijacks levodopa is catechol-O-methyl-transferase or COMT for short. If COMT is inhibited, more levodopa can reach the brain's motor control system. The principle is almost identical to that operating with DDIs such as carbidopa, which have been packaged with levodopa for about forty years. The COMT inhibitors are used by people who develop motor fluctuations with carbidopa/levodopa and need an additional enzyme inhibitor in their medication.

The MAO-B inhibitors, such as selegiline (Eldepryl) and rasagiline (Azilect), prevent the enzyme monoamine oxidase type B from breaking down dopamine in the brain itself and thus increase the dopamine level in the brain and, in theory, help relieve Parkinson's symptoms. MAO-B inhibitors, which function only inside the brain, have less of a symptomatic effect than COMT inhibitors.

COMT Inhibitors. Approved by the FDA in 1998, the first COMT inhibitor was *tolcapone* (Tasmar). A second COMT inhibitor, *entacapone* (Comtan), was approved by the FDA in late 1999. The COMT inhibitors manipulate a biochemical pathway that, before 1998, had not been targeted in the treatment of Parkinson's disease. Patients may experience particular benefit with combination therapy that includes carbidopa/levodopa, a dopamine agonist, and a COMT inhibitor. In fact, a triple combination drug—carbidopa/entacapone/levodopa (Stalevo)—has been marketed for convenience.

COMT inhibitors are particularly helpful for people who have motor fluctuations. As discussed earlier, motor fluctuations occur as the level of dopamine in the brain fluctuates. If the brain has adequate dopamine, people are "on" and can move almost normally; if it does not, they become increasingly slow and stiff and may become frozen. Any medication that results in more dopamine being delivered to the brain for a longer time should prolong the "on" time and reduce the "off" time, and COMT inhibitors have been shown to be effective in doing this.

Tolcapone and entacapone have very simple dosing schedules. Because it is not necessary to start with a low dose and increase slowly, an effective dose can be started on the first day for both these medications. For this reason, both are easier to use than the dopamine agonists. Tolcapone is taken three times a day. Entacapone is a shorter-acting drug and is given with every dose of carbidopa/levodopa up to ten times a day.

Both COMT inhibitors may have some troubling side effects, however. Some are the same side effects produced by most dopamine-stimulating drugs: dizziness, nausea, fatigue, orthostatic hypotension, dyskinesia, and hallucinations. Side effects are often manageable by reducing the levodopa dosage.

COMT inhibitors may pose particular problems for people who have trouble with dyskinesia. If these involuntary movements become worse at the peak of the levodopa dose, the person is reacting to increased stimulation to the dopamine system. Because COMT inhibitors increase the available dopamine, adding it to a drug regimen is likely to increase the frequency and severity of any dyskinesia. One solution may be to reduce the levodopa dosage, usually by about 20 to 25 percent, when adding the COMT inhibitor (this is generally done as a preventative measure if the patient already has bothersome dyskinesias when COMT inhibitors are being started). When the right balance is achieved, people generally experience improved "on" time with little worsening of the dyskinesia.

Some side effects of COMT inhibitors require serious attention. The non-life-threatening one is diarrhea: approximately one month after beginning treatment, 5 to 10 percent of patients taking a COMT inhibitor develop diarrhea. This usually means the drug must be discontinued. Not all diarrhea caused by COMT inhibitors is so serious, however, and if it is mild, the drug can be continued. You should tell your physician if you have diarrhea after starting a COMT inhibitor.

The more serious complication is the possibility of liver malfunction. We know that 2 to 3 percent of people taking tolcapone (Tasmar) develop elevated blood levels of enzymes called transaminases, which indicates a disturbance of liver function. Some people develop severe liver damage with tolcapone. This rare but serious toxicity to the liver has led the FDA to issue a severe warning about the use of tolcapone. It is to be prescribed only for people who have advanced Parkinson's after other antiparkinson medications have been used; it should be tried for three weeks, then if no benefit is noted by this time, it should be stopped. Anyone who takes Tasmar must sign a consent form indicating they are aware of the risk of severe liver failure and death.

In early 2006, the FDA, after studying the use of tolcapone in many people who have Parkinson's disease, eased the restrictions on its use. Someone planning to take tolcapone must have liver function tests before starting the drug and then be closely monitored for liver function every two to four weeks for the first six months. After six months of treatment, the doctor determines whether continued liver function testing is necessary. The hope is that the frequent liver tests will prevent toxic damage to the liver by alerting the doctor to the first signs of damage, so tolcapone can be stopped immediately. This approach may be working. In the United States since the new regulations requiring liver monitoring, no deaths due to Tasmar use have been reported. (In Canada and Europe, Tasmar was taken off the market, but it has recently been reinstated in Europe.)

Entacapone does not have these liver toxicity problems, and liver monitoring is not necessary for people using this drug. If COMT inhibitors are to be prescribed, entacapone should be used first. It is worth noting, however, that if a person has had trouble with motor fluctuations and has unsuccessfully tried using entacapone, she or he might want to consider trying tolcapone, even with the liver function monitoring. Tolcapone is very useful for many people and the hope is that further use of this drug will demonstrate that the liver toxicity is extremely rare; if this is so, the close monitoring of tolcapone may be relaxed.

MAO Inhibitors. MAO inhibitors have been available longer than COMT inhibitors, a number of them having been developed as antidepressants. The MAO system of enzymes is divided into subsidiary systems called MAO-A and MAO-B. The MAO-A inhibitors and the nonselective MAO inhibitors—those that inhibit either the MAO-A or the MAO-B system—relieve depression apparently by increasing the amount of dopamine and norepinephrine in the brain.

People taking the older nonselective MAO inhibitors (e.g., pargyline) must avoid eating certain foods in order to prevent the so-called cheese effect. When combined with the MAO-A inhibitors or the nonselective MAO inhibitors, a compound called *tyramine,* common in aged cheese, red wines, and beer, can be transformed into a chemical that can elevate blood pressure to dangerously high levels. This same problem also occurs if these MAO inhibitors are given with levodopa, so they are generally not used in treating Parkinson's disease and should never be given to a person taking levodopa.

Fortunately for people who have Parkinson's, the MAO-B inhibitors, such as *selegiline* (Eldepryl) and *rasagiline* (Azilect), do not produce the cheese effect in the doses (5 to 10 milligrams a day for selegiline; 1 milligram a day for rasagiline) used to treat Parkinson's, and the dietary restrictions do not apply. Selegiline is used primarily to smooth out the motor performance of people who have moderate to advanced disease who are having difficulties with motor fluctuations. Its effects are very mild and sometimes cannot be perceived by the person taking it or by the doctor.

A hypothesis that selegiline might protect against the degeneration occurring in Parkinson's disease has not been proved by research. Finding an agent that would halt or slow the progression of Parkinson's has been something of a Holy Grail. Even a small reduction in the progression of Parkinson's disease might add years to a person's ability to enjoy life unhindered by Parkinson's-related disability or medication.

The idea that selegiline might be such a drug stemmed from research on MPTP, the drug that was illegally and mistakenly prepared then intravenously self-administered, causing rapid development of symptoms of advanced parkinsonism (see Chapter 9). Used in animal experiments, MPTP destroyed the cells of the substantia nigra in a way so similar to Parkinson's that it provided an excellent model for Parkinson's disease research.

Research showed that inhibiting the function of MAO prevented MPTP-induced parkinsonism in animals. Scientists hypothesized that Parkinson's might be caused by some unknown environmental toxin that works in a way similar to MPTP, or that in breaking down dopamine, MAO might produce toxic by-products that could contribute to the nerve cell loss in Parkinson's. If either or both of these hypotheses were true, perhaps an MAO inhibitor could prevent the progressive neuronal damage in Parkinson's disease.

In search of a neuroprotective agent, the Parkinson Study Group (PSG), a consortium of Parkinson's investigators from across North

America, enrolled patients with very early symptoms of Parkinson's in a study to monitor the progression of their disease. This large-scale study was known as the DATATOP (*Deprenyl and Tocopherol Antioxidative Therapy of Parkinson's*) trial. The DATATOP trial was designed to study people who have early Parkinson's disease who would not require levodopa for several years, to determine whether or not selegiline (also known as deprenyl) or high doses of vitamin E (also known as tocopherol) could slow the progression of Parkinson's. (Vitamin E, an antioxidant, was included because it is believed to protect cells from damage due to toxins known as free radicals.)

Study participants were divided into four groups: one group received selegiline, one received vitamin E, one received both selegiline and vitamin E, and one received a placebo (sugar pill). People were carefully observed during the trial, and the trial for each person ended when his or her symptoms became serious enough to require levodopa therapy. Researchers kept track of how long it took before participants required levodopa therapy.

The results, reported in the *New England Journal of Medicine,* showed that people who received 2,000 units of vitamin E daily did no better than those who received the placebo, which ruled out vitamin E as a protective agent. The selegiline group, though, clearly did better than the placebo group, going longer before they needed levodopa. This part of the study leaves us with a controversy.

Other scientific research reported that selegiline at the level used in the DATATOP trial did not improve Parkinson's symptoms, but, as was clear from the DATATOP study, for some people selegiline was indeed able to produce some symptomatic relief of tremor, slowness, or rigidity. How are we to make sense of these conflicting conclusions? Did the patients taking selegiline require levodopa later than those not taking selegiline because this drug slowed down the underlying disease progression, or because they were already taking a medication (selegiline) with mildly beneficial symptomatic effects? To further muddy the interpretative waters, at the same time that the DATATOP results were reported, the FDA approved the use of selegiline for people who have moderate to advanced Parkinson's, so the drug was available for physicians to prescribe.

All these events caused considerable confusion among clinical researchers, neurologists, and patients and their families. It seemed that the FDA had approved selegiline because it was mildly effective in relieving symptoms, yet the *New England Journal* had reported that it might delay the need for levodopa. Hopes were high for neuroprotection, and many physicians prescribed selegiline for people who have Parkinson's who wanted to try this new drug.

With time, the initial excitement gave way to disappointment as the long-term follow-up data from the DATATOP trial were less and less encouraging. The PSG reported that although initial use of selegiline delayed levodopa use, the drug didn't appear to have any neuroprotective effect. Also, the drug didn't delay the appearance of levodopa side effects such as motor fluctuations or dyskinesia. On the other hand, a long-term study from Sweden did provide some supportive evidence for a disease modifying effect (a term sometimes used interchangeably with *neuroprotection,* although there are important differences) of selegiline.

THE DATATOP STUDY was just one in a series of neuroprotective trials that used the MPTP animal model of Parkinson's as the scientific basis for the trial. In other words, the experimental (neuroprotective) drugs had been shown in animal models to slow or lessen the damage to dopamine cells that MPTP caused. The failure of so many trials based on this model is what has called the future usefulness of the MPTP Parkinson model into question.

Even today, the controversy about the role of selegiline in Parkinson's disease continues. Some neurologists continue to believe that selegiline has a mild neuroprotective effect, while others believe it has solely a mild symptomatic effect. What both camps do agree on is that the effects of selegiline, whether neuroprotective or symptomatic, are mild. Its effects are less potent than the effects of most other Parkinson's medications, and many patients report few noticeable changes in their symptoms when they start or stop taking selegiline.

The weight of the evidence suggests that selegiline does not provide neuroprotection for people who have early, moderate, or advanced Parkinson's disease. The use of selegiline should be reserved for those who require it as a symptomatic drug to enhance dopamine's effects in the early stages of the disease or to improve motor fluctuations in later stages.

You may have heard reports that use of selegiline might be associated with increased mortality. This concern is related to a study from the United Kingdom reported in the *British Medical Journal*. The study found that the death rate among people taking levodopa plus selegiline was considerably higher than that among people taking levodopa alone. Although this result is extremely disturbing, it has not been corroborated in several other large patient series, and generally the possibility of increased mortality among selegiline users is considered highly unlikely. Numerous flaws were noted in the U.K. study. Subsequently, the DATATOP patient groups were thoroughly analyzed and no evidence of increased mortality was found among the selegiline users.

A form of selegiline (Zydis Selegiline or Zelapar) has been introduced for the treatment of Parkinson's disease. The tablet of Zelapar is placed in the mouth, and it dissolves rapidly without water. The drug is absorbed into the body through the lining of the mouth, rather than through the stomach. This may improve its usefulness in alleviating symptoms of Parkinson's disease and lowers the dose needed by avoiding early metabolism by the liver.

Rasagiline (Azilect) is a newer MAO-B inhibitor that has been used in early and moderate Parkinson's with success. In early Parkinson's it has beneficial effects on the motor symptoms, and in moderate to advanced Parkinson's it helps reduce motor fluctuations and results in more "on" time. In fact, in one large study, rasagiline was comparable to entacapone in reducing motor fluctuations.

In a variety of animal models, including models of Parkinson's, stroke, and head trauma, there are reports that rasagiline can protect neurons in the brain. Of course, one of the repeated problems in Parkinson's research is the success of a drug in an animal model but failure of the drug in people who have Parkinson's. Rasagiline is currently being promoted as a neuroprotective drug, but no clear evidence or proof exists that it really slows the progression of Parkinson's.

One very interesting clinical research trial, again conducted by the PSG, examined the effectiveness of rasagiline in people who have early Parkinson's. This trial divided people into three groups: those taking rasagiline, 1 milligram a day for six months; those taking rasagiline, 2 milligrams a day for six months; and those taking a placebo (sugar pill) each day for six months. Not surprisingly, at the end of six months, the groups that had received 1 or 2 milligrams of rasagiline a day had improved motor symptoms (tremor, rigidity, and bradykinesia) compared with those in the placebo group. During the second six months of the study, the groups receiving 1 or 2 milligrams a day continued on their same rasagiline dose, and the placebo group started taking 2 milligrams a day. The Parkinson's scores were again evaluated six months later, or twelve months after the start of the entire research trial. Starting rasagiline in one group after six months of placebo is an example of a *delayed start* trial (see Chapter 11).

Delayed start trials are a new method for trying to establish whether a particular drug is neuroprotective. One of the big problems in clinical research on Parkinson's is that if a drug relieves symptoms, then it is impossible to know whether that same drug has any neuroprotective effect. This is the problem we described earlier concerning the DATA-TOP trial of selegiline.

In the delayed start trial of rasagiline, there was some evidence that people who have early Parkinson's were better off starting treatment earlier rather than delaying for six months. In other words, there was less worsening of Parkinson's scores for the patients who took rasagiline for twelve months than for those who took placebo for six months followed by six months of rasagiline. This was an intriguing finding that encouraged the subsequent delayed-start ADAGIO study that was discussed in Chapter 11, which unfortunately has not provided us with a definitive answer. Much additional research needs to be conducted before we can be sure that these results really represent neuroprotection or an actual modification of the disease process. There are many alternative explanations of why starting medications earlier rather than later might potentially affect outcome.

Understandably, there continues to be great interest in neuroprotection, and several new agents are under study that may one day be capable of slowing disease progression. The discovery of a true neuroprotective agent for use in Parkinson's disease will be a milestone in the therapy of this disease.

Anticholinergics and Amantadine

The anticholinergic drugs and amantadine have a long and honorable history in the treatment of Parkinson's disease. They are still useful in early Parkinson's and are sometimes helpful in alleviating symptoms for advanced disease. They are not as effective in moderate Parkinson's as the major drugs that manipulate the dopamine system, and they have substantial side effects. If these drugs are used, they must be started at the lowest possible dose, introduced slowly, and increased gradually.

Anticholinergics. Made from the herb belladonna, the belladonna alkaloids were the major therapy for the symptoms of Parkinson's disease during the late nineteenth and early twentieth centuries. Synthetic anticholinergic medications replaced belladonna alkaloids in the 1950s and remained the major category of drugs for treatment of Parkinson's until the introduction of levodopa in the late 1960s. Even today, these medications are used to help control tremor and drooling. They are not as useful as other drugs in relieving rigidity, slowness, or walking problems.

As noted in Chapter 11, the acetylcholine and dopamine neurotransmitter systems are finely balanced, and because Parkinson's depletes the dopamine system, people who have Parkinson's disease have an excess of acetylcholine activity. Anticholinergic drugs work by partially blocking the acetylcholine system and bringing the two neurotransmitter systems back into balance, thus relieving symptoms.

The anticholinergic medications include a wide variety of compounds, such as trihexyphenidyl (Artane), benztropine (Cogentin), procyclidine (Kemadrin), ethopropazine (Parsitan, Parsidol), and biperiden (Akineton). They are used mainly to reduce the resting tremor of Parkinson's disease. Also, a low dose of an anticholinergic medication such as Artane, Cogentin, or Parsitan can be helpful for a person who has difficulty with drooling or with controlling saliva.

A number of side effects are associated with these drugs, limiting their use, although some people can take an effective dose without any apparent problem. Anticholinergics may cause sedation, constipation, blurred vision, and, most troubling, urinary retention (men with enlargement of the prostate should avoid anticholinergics) and cognitive impairment (problems with thinking and memory). Some people taking these drugs describe feeling mentally dull, forgetful, less attentive, and unable to concentrate. Older people may be particularly susceptible to the drug's effects on their memory and thinking, and they may even become confused and disoriented.

Because anticholinergic medications are primarily helpful for tremor, and because they have these adverse side effects, many people who have Parkinson's never use them. These drugs are rarely appropriate for elderly people and are almost never used for people who have had problems with memory or mental function. Some people are uncomfortable with the mouth dryness, constipation, or visual blurring, and these side effects also keep them from using anticholinergics.

When anticholinergics are to be discontinued after an individual has been taking them for a long time, they should be decreased slowly, never stopped abruptly. Discontinuing them suddenly can cause a "rebound" effect, a temporary worsening of symptoms. This applies to symptoms other than tremor, even though anticholinergics are not very useful in relieving these other symptoms in the first place. This rebound may last for days, occasionally extending to weeks, until the brain has time to readjust its chemical balance.

Amantadine. Amantadine (Symmetrel) has been used to treat Parkinson's disease for decades. Its antiparkinson effects were first recognized when people who have Parkinson's took it for a different purpose (to prevent influenza) and reported to their neurologists that their parkinsonian symptoms had improved. This led to studies demonstrating that amantadine does indeed have the ability to relieve the slowness and rigidity of Parkinson's disease.

There are several hypotheses on why amantadine is effective in Parkinson's disease. It may interfere with the reuptake of dopamine or it may promote the release of dopamine. Either of these mechanisms would have the effect of increasing the availability of dopamine in the brain. Given that Parkinson's is primarily a dopamine deficiency problem, any drug that enhances dopamine in the brain will tend to relieve its symptoms. Amantadine also has anticholinergic effects. Recent studies on amantadine have indicated that it affects the glutamate system, and this finding may indeed account for the majority of the drug's clinical effects; *glutamate* is another important neurotransmitter in the brain that may be involved in parkinsonian symptoms.

Amantadine is used most often in early Parkinson's disease to relieve mild stiffness, slowness, and minor gait abnormalities. Although you may read that its usefulness lasts only ten to twelve weeks, some people benefit from amantadine for much longer. Recently there has been interest in the use of amantadine for people who have more advanced disease who are having difficulty with motor fluctuations, dyskinesia, and more severe gait problems. Amantadine reduces the severity of dyskinesia in some but not all people. No adequate study of amantadine for the advanced stage of Parkinson's has been conducted; however, we have prescribed amantadine in this way, to the benefit of many people.

Amantadine has some potential adverse effects. It should not be used by people whose kidneys are not functioning well. Amantadine is eliminated from the body by the kidneys, and people who have poor kidney function may have a toxic buildup of the drug. Like all medications for Parkinson's disease, even for patients with perfectly normal kidney function, amantadine can cause personality changes, feelings of fogginess, unexplained malaise, forgetfulness, and occasionally hallucinations and confusion. All the cognitive and personality changes induced by amantadine can be eliminated by stopping the medication.

Amantadine also has some relatively minor side effects. It may produce a skin reaction known as *livedo reticularis,* which typically has a blotchy or mottled, red, streaky pattern. This may be unsightly but it is not dangerous. When the amantadine is discontinued, the skin changes disappear over several months. Amantadine can also cause the ankles to swell, and this occasionally causes mild discomfort with a feeling of tightness in the affected area. But if a person's Parkinson's symptoms are substantially relieved by amantadine, neither livedo reticularis nor swelling of the ankles is generally reason enough to stop the drug.

Drugs for the Other Symptoms of Parkinson's

Many people who have Parkinson's need medications to relieve symptoms other than the characteristic symptoms of tremor, rigidity, slowness, and problems with walking and balance. As noted in earlier chapters, there is evidence that Parkinson's itself can cause some depression, anxiety, sleep disruption, cognitive impairment, muscle cramps, and constipation. Some of these problems can be handled by making changes in lifestyle, but if that does not work, or if these other symptoms have become severe, drugs are available to help.

Depression

In Parkinson's disease, the brain systems that degenerate include some parts of the brain involved in emotion, so depression may be an effect of the disease itself, or a sign of difficulty with adjustment to chronic symptoms, or a combination of both. (The symptoms of depression are described in Chapters 3 and 6.) If depression is interfering with daily functioning, it should be treated.

A number of medications are frequently successful in treating depression. Some of the older antidepressant medications, such as the *tricyclic antidepressants* (TCAs), remain useful in Parkinson's disease. Amitriptyline (Elavil) and nortriptyline (Pamelor) are examples of TCAs. These drugs tend to sedate people, so they can also help people who have sleep disturbances. The side effects include dry mouth and excessive sleepiness, and there could be changes in behavior such as memory dysfunction or confusion. If you are taking these medications and have any adverse effects, ask your doctor about stopping the medication. Its effects are reversible.

Newer antidepressants, called *selective serotonin reuptake inhibitors* (SSRIs), are also effective in relieving the depression of Parkinson's disease. Examples of these drugs are fluoxetine (Prozac), sertraline (Zoloft), escitalopram (Lexapro), duloxetine (Cymbalta), and paroxetine (Paxil). The SSRIs may be easier to take and better tolerated. They also may relieve anxiety. Venlafaxine (Effexor) is a combination serotonin and norepinephrine reuptake inhibitor that is generally well tolerated and effective for depression in people who have Parkinson's disease.

Determining which antidepressants work for which people is not easy. Although very few studies have compared different antidepressants to determine which are the best for depression or anxiety in Parkinson's, a clinical trial comparing the antidepressant effects of Paxil, Effexor, and placebo in Parkinson's disease showed that both Paxil and Effexor were superior to placebo. Finding the right medication requires patience, because most of these medications require a four- to six-week period to achieve their full effect. If one drug does not work, it is important to try another. Failure of one drug to relieve symptoms does not mean one of the other drugs won't work.

Also, antidepressants may interact with other drugs. Both TCAs and the SSRI antidepressants can be taken with all the antiparkinson medications, but some precautions are important. Some pills are not just TCAs or SSRIs; they may combine a TCA such as amitriptyline with a major tranquilizer such as perphenazine. These combinations (e.g., Triavil) should never be used by people who have Parkinson's. The perphenazine will make Parkinson's symptoms worse. Another antidepressant, amoxapine (Asendin), has similar effects and should not be used by people who have Parkinson's.

There have been reports of SSRIs worsening the signs of Parkinson's disease or causing symptoms of parkinsonism in people who had no previous symptoms. In our experience this is a rare occurrence and is not a reason for a depressed person who has Parkinson's to avoid SSRIs. If you are taking an SSRI, it *is* important to monitor your symptoms and tell your physician if your symptoms increase when you start the drug.

The FDA has issued a warning about the use of SSRI antidepressants in combination with selegiline. The warning is based on a few reports suggesting that the combination of an SSRI such as sertraline (Zoloft) or paroxetine (Paxil) and an MAO inhibitor such as selegiline (Eldepryl) may result in a group of symptoms called the *serotonin syndrome*. The syndrome is characterized by anxiety, agitation, rigidity, and elevated temperature. Because this combination of medications is commonly used, the FDA warning caused considerable concern among neurologists and persons who have Parkinson's.

To check on the warning's validity, a survey was done of Parkinson's disease specialists who treat large numbers of people. Physicians reported very few cases of serotonin syndrome in their patients. This survey provided little evidence to support the discontinuation of selegiline (Eldepryl) combined with an SSRI. Despite the FDA warning, we continue to prescribe this combination when we think both medications are clearly warranted.

If these two medications—selegiline and an SSRI—have been prescribed together for you, discuss the issue with your physician.

Anxiety

People who have Parkinson's may become anxious, develop social phobias, or have panic attacks. The anxiety is believed to be a result of both the biochemical changes in the brain and the stress of coping with Parkinson's symptoms. (See Chapters 5 and 6 for more details.)

The SSRIs are frequently effective in alleviating anxiety. People can take them once a day to reduce feelings of anxiety throughout the day.

Many doctors prescribe drugs classified as *anxiolytics* for people who complain of nervousness. The most common are the *benzodiazepines*, including diazepam (Valium), lorazepam (Ativan), and alprazolam (Xanax). Benzodiazepines are taken at the time a person feels anxious. They may also be helpful as muscle relaxants or to induce sleep. Benzodiazepines have a major disadvantage: regular usage results in both tolerance to the drug's effects and physical dependence on the drug. *Tolerance* means that when people take the medication regularly, after some time they may require increased dosages to obtain the same effect. *Physical dependence* means that if benzodiazepines have been used for months, they cannot be discontinued abruptly. The dosage must be reduced slowly and gradually, before stopping. Side effects of benzodiazepines include sleepiness, forgetfulness, and mild confusion. These drugs should be used judiciously.

Sleep Disruption

Sleep disruption (discussed in Chapter 4) is common among people who have Parkinson's. A physician can usually give patients an idea of whether their sleep disruption is related to Parkinson's or is simply fairly typical for someone of their age (healthy older people often sleep fewer hours at night and nap during the day). People sometimes can handle sleep disruption by changing habits (for suggestions, see Chapter 4). Sometimes the sleep problems are caused by drugs; other times, they are caused by inadequate medication to treat nighttime Parkinson's symptoms. If tremor, rigidity, and slowness are problems at night, the person may benefit from taking a carbidopa/levodopa dose at night or using a long-acting Parkinson's medication such as Sinemet CR, the controlled-release carbidopa/levodopa preparation.

Antiparkinson medications, particularly carbidopa/levodopa and the dopamine receptor agonists, may have a sedating effect, causing daytime sleepiness. If these drugs are needed to control serious tremor, rigidity, slowness, and walking problems to allow ease of movement during the day, the person is caught in a dilemma. Sometimes it is possible to adjust dosages or medication schedules or try different antiparkinson drugs. Stimulants, such as amphetamines or methylphenidate (Ritalin), are rarely effective. Excessive daytime sleepiness can sometimes be helped with the use of modafinil (Provigil).

As we've noted in earlier chapters, some people are mistakenly diagnosed as having Parkinson's. Atypical Parkinson's syndromes (see Chapter 10) often fail to respond to carbidopa/levodopa, and people who have these disorders may be sedated by a medication that is not helping them in any way. To check this, they may need to stop the medication gradually. If they become alert and their motor symptoms do not become worse, they probably do not have true Parkinson's disease.

Many other commonly prescribed medications can contribute to excessive daytime sleepiness: sleeping pills used at bedtime, as well as drugs for anxiety, depression, muscle spasms, pain, and urinary incontinence. For people who are excessively sleepy in the daytime, attempting to reduce or eliminate these medications makes good sense.

We consider lifestyle changes the preferred first line of defense against sleep disruption. We are cautious about prescribing any sedatives to help people who have Parkinson's fall asleep. Parkinson's patients are already taking medications that affect their brain function, and sleep medication can have long-lasting effects. Particularly for older individuals or people who have preexisting cognitive disturbances, adding any medications that dull the mind may cause confusion and disorientation during the night and even the next day.

That said, when lifestyle approaches—such as adequate exercise and avoiding caffeine and daytime naps—are not adequate, we sometimes prescribe sedatives and sleep medications. A broad range of choices is available, including medications specifically indicated for insomnia, such as temazepam (Restoril) or zolpidem (Ambien), and medications that have sedating qualities although they are indicated for other problems, such as depression or anxiety—for example, amitriptyline (Elavil), trazodone (Desyrel), and diazepam (Valium). Such medications should not be used routinely but only when necessary and then in the lowest possible effective dosage.

Sleep Attacks

Reports have described excessive daytime sleepiness and what is called *sleep attacks* due to the dopamine agonists pramipexole and ropinerole. This has stimulated considerable study and it is now clear that excessive sleepiness even to the point of falling asleep while driving can occur with most antiparkinson drugs. It is not clear whether this is more common with specific agonists. Patients and physicians need to be aware of this problem to monitor any excessive sleepiness that occurs while a patient is taking these drugs and adjust activities, particularly driving, accordingly. Some patients without excessive daytime sleepiness experience nighttime insomnia in response to dopamine agonists—particularly, in our experience, with pramipexole.

Psychotic Symptoms

When a person loses the ability to distinguish reality from dreams or hallucinations, physicians diagnose this as *psychotic behavior.* In people who have Parkinson's disease, psychosis is almost always drug related. People may insist that the children, strangers, animals, and insects they "see" are real. They may insist that their spouse is having an affair, stealing from them, poisoning them, or conspiring against them. They may also experience severe confusion or mania and act belligerently or aggressively.

The management of levodopa-related psychosis is complicated. The behavioral abnormalities can be improved by reducing the dose of antiparkinson medications, including carbidopa/levodopa, or omitting certain medications altogether. However, when the amount of antiparkinson medications is reduced, the underlying parkinsonian symptoms often become more prominent. Fortunately, we have many approaches to solving this problem, including carefully reducing the dosage of certain medications, discontinuing some medications, or adding atypical antipsychotic agents such as quetiapine (Seroquel) or clozapine (Clozaril). Atypical antipsychotics can suppress psychotic symptoms but are less likely to make parkinsonism worse than the typical antipsychotics. Anyone taking clozapine needs to have frequent blood tests because of the risk of a reduced white blood cell count. This drug should be administered only by physicians who are experienced with the medication and the procedures involved in its administration. Clozapine is the most effective agent for the management of psychosis in people who have Parkinson's disease that cannot be adequately handled by changes in antiparkinson medications. Due to the inconvenience caused by need for blood monitoring, most physicians will give a trial of quetiapine first before turning to clozapine; quetiapine, however, is very definitely the less effective of the two drugs for this problem. Patients and families should be reassured that when clozapine is appropriately monitored with regular blood counts (as it has to be for the patient to obtain the drug) it is an extremely safe drug and no cases of permanent bone marrow damage have occurred in patients undergoing regular monitoring.

Cognitive Impairment

As discussed in Chapter 6, thinking and memory problems are not uncommon, particularly in patients with long-standing Parkinson's disease. Other causes for these symptoms need to be excluded, including confusion induced by medications or other illnesses such as infections and difficulty concentrating due to depression or anxiety. When cognitive impairment and dementia occur as part of the primary illness this is usually due to the Parkinson's disease process affecting brain regions responsible for higher cognitive function as well as additional brain changes similar to those seen in Alzheimer's disease. Cognitive enhancing drugs have been developed and marketed for Alzheimer's disease. The commonest mechanism of action of these drugs is the enhancement of levels of the brain neurotransmitter acetylcholine by blocking its enzymatic breakdown. As mentioned earlier in this chapter, anticholinergics (drugs that block the action of acetylcholine) are sometimes used to treat the symptoms of Parkinson's disease (particularly tremor); the confusion and memory loss that can sometimes occur as side effects of these drugs relate to their action outside the basal ganglia, in the brain cortical regions involved in memory. Reduced levels of acetylcholine in these regions are thought to partially explain cognitive disturbances in Alzheimer's disease. Interestingly, these levels may be even lower in Parkinson's disease than in Alzheimer's. For this reason, drugs developed initially for use in Alzheimer's disease can sometimes provide considerable benefit to patients with Parkinson-related cognitive dysfunction. Donepezil (Aricept), rivastigmine (Exelon), and galantamine (Reminyl) are the three available cholinesterase inhibitors released for the treatment of Alzheimer's disease. Rivastigmine has the best available evidence in the medical literature supporting its use in Parkinson's disease–related dementia while the evidence for efficacy of donepezil and galantamine is less strong. Gastrointestinal side effects such as nausea, vomiting, and diarrhea are not uncommon with these drugs. The use of the skin patch formulation of rivastigmine may be better tolerated with respect to these side effects. Because these drugs increase acetylcholine in the basal ganglia they can aggravate rest tremor (i.e., opposite to the effects of anticholinergic drugs), and this may be a reason for having to stop these drugs. Memantine is another "cognitive enhancing" agent marketed for Alzheimer's disease. This drug works by blocking glutamate N-methyl D-aspartate (NMDA) receptors in the brain. This too can be used in Parkinson's related dementia although its beneficial effects have not been clearly proven.

Muscle Cramps

Many people who have Parkinson's ask for muscle relaxants to relieve the stiff and rigid feeling they experience in the course of the day. However, the traditional muscle relaxants do not provide much relief because the problem is not in the muscles but in the muscle control system. Also, people who have Parkinson's frequently are taking numerous drugs already, so generally it is not a good idea to unnecessarily add to their burden of medication.

For dystonic muscle spasm, baclofen (Lioresal), a special type of muscle relaxant, may be helpful both at bedtime and intermittently throughout the day, but we prefer to adjust the levels of other antiparkinson medication, as described in Chapter 4. Dystonic cramps occur particularly in the early morning, when dopamine levels in the brain are low following a long night without medication. Sometimes they occur intermittently when individual doses wear off during the day. Dystonic spasms that occur during the night or in the early morning can often be eliminated by taking Sinemet CR at bedtime. If the spasms occur exclusively after waking at the same time every morning, another successful approach is to set the alarm for one or two hours earlier, take a dose of regular carbidopa/levodopa at the bedside, and go back to sleep until the usual waking time. By then the levels of brain dopamine are usually high enough to prevent the dystonic spasm.

Constipation

Constipation is without question the most common alteration of bowel habits in people who have Parkinson's, perhaps because of the many potential causes of constipation: normal aging, the Parkinson's degeneration of motor control of muscles in the lower digestive tract, increased sedentary habits, and antiparkinson medications (see Chapter 4).

Again, the first and best defense is lifestyle changes. People should drink five to six glasses of water a day, increase the amount of roughage (fiber) in their diets, and exercise to keep the intestinal muscles moving. Emptying the bowels at the same time each day is helpful. Typically, morning works well, and people can encourage regular movements by eating a breakfast that includes fiber and prunes and then going for a walk.

If increased fluid intake and increased roughage in the diet are not adequate to take care of the problem, people can take fiber-rich preparations such as Metamucil or Konsyl and stool softeners such as Colace. The osmotic laxative polyethylene glycol (Miralax) can also be very useful. Stronger medications such as lactulose syrup, Dulcolax tablets/suppositories, milk of magnesia, or enemas may or may not be needed. Severe constipation can be a medical emergency and on rare occasion can lead to bowel obstruction.

OVER THE PAST THREE DECADES, levodopa has restored the function of countless people who have Parkinson's disease around the world. It is the single most effective drug in the treatment of moderate to advanced Parkinson's. Until a treatment is developed to protect neurons from damage, levodopa is likely to remain the mainstay of Parkinson's disease treatment. In this chapter, we have described how levodopa can be used with other drugs to achieve the best control of symptoms. In Chapters 14 and 15 we consider other approaches to controlling symptoms, then in Chapter 16 we turn to a consideration of surgical therapies.

CHAPTER 14

Exercise and
Rehabilitation Therapy

- *Is exercise helpful for the symptoms of Parkinson's disease?*
- *What is the best exercise regimen?*
- *How can exercise or rehabilitation therapy help?*
- *When is the right time to visit a rehabilitation therapist?*

It is only recently that exercise has been recognized as an important part of the management of Parkinson's disease. This change in the way we think of exercise is illustrated by the development of this new chapter devoted solely to the topic of exercise in this edition of our book. For many people, the benefits of exercise seem obvious and intuitive, so why has this taken so long? The answer is likely to be a combination of factors including less funding for research in nonpharmacologic approaches to treatment and less medical training in the use of exercise modalities. But the tide has turned—now many neurologists proudly describe that they recommend exercise for all of their patients with Parkinson's disease, and more opportunities for physical activity for people who have Parkinson's are developed each year, ranging from basic fitness to yoga, tai chi, or dance. Although still relatively limited, funding options for research in exercise and rehabilitation training are increasing, along with a steady increase in our knowledge and understanding. In fact, 90 percent of the research in exercise and rehabilitation in Parkinson's has been performed in the last decade.

What Is the Difference between Exercise and Rehabilitation Therapy?

For the purpose of this chapter, we will use "rehabilitation" to refer to a training program performed under the guidance of a licensed rehabilitation therapist, and we will use "exercise" to refer to physical activity that is performed in a routine manner in a community (nonmedical) setting. Rehabilitation includes physical therapy (PT), occupational therapy (OT), and speech therapy (ST). These types of therapy are generally covered by health insurance and require a physician's order. Speech therapists focus on problems with speech and swallowing. Speech problems in Parkinson's include low volume of the voice (hypophonia), slurred speech, or stuttering. Speech therapists evaluate the swallowing mechanism with swallowing studies and provide guidance on approaches that ease swallowing difficulty (dysphagia). Occupational therapists focus on evaluating your ability to perform daily activities independently. These "activities of daily living" (ADLs) include basic tasks like bathing, dressing, eating, and toileting. The so-called instrumental activities of daily living (IADLs) are more complex and include tasks like preparing meals, shopping, traveling, and managing medications. Occupational therapists provide guidance on how best to accomplish your everyday activities even when Parkinson's symptoms intervene. Physical therapists focus on general mobility, strength, and range of motion. Typical reasons for visiting a physical therapist include walking problems, falls, and general "deconditioning" (poor endurance and fitness).

Based on the main problems identified during a routine office visit, your physician may decide that you will benefit from evaluation and treatment by physical, occupational, and/or speech therapy. Identifying the "right" timing for rehabilitation therapy can be challenging and requires good communication between the physician and the person who has Parkinson's. If you notice that your risk of falling has increased or that you need more assistance with your daily activities or that you are having new problems with swallowing, discuss these issues with your physician and ask whether this is a good time to visit a physical, occupational, or speech therapist. Rehabilitation therapists have a varied range of experience with Parkinson's disease, and there are relatively few therapists who specialize in Parkinson's. In addition, the approaches used by physical and occupational therapists are quite variable. The optimum rehabilitation therapy for people who have Parkinson's is provided by therapists who are highly experienced in Parkinson's and who use techniques based on evidence from successful clinical trials. But this can be hard to find. It is worthwhile to "shop around" to find a therapist who cares regularly for people who have Parkinson's.

Physical therapists can help you develop an exercise regimen that is safe and appropriate for your fitness and level of symptoms. People who have early Parkinson's who are reasonably fit may use an exercise trainer for this purpose. A therapist is particularly helpful for people who have been sedentary or who have Parkinson's symptoms that may interfere with their ability to perform certain types of exercise. In this situation, it is important to identify an exercise routine that is safe yet challenging based on the individual's level of fitness.

"I already get plenty of exercise"

Some people who have Parkinson's tell us that they don't need an exercise program because they "already get plenty of exercise" in their daily activities. They often say that they are already on their feet all day because they are watching their kids or grandkids, or they have a busy workday or do a lot of housekeeping. But the effort in your daily activities is not equivalent to an exercise program. Daily activities generally involve a lot of stopping and starting movements, while aerobic exercise involves steady exercise that keeps your heart rate elevated over a period of time. Also, daily activities generally involve certain movements and muscle groups as you perform similar movements repetitively (lifting packages, walking the dog, cleaning the dishes), while a good exercise routine involves a combination of different types of exercise that train the upper and lower body, the trunk, and cardiovascular fitness.

What Have We Learned from Studies of Exercise and Rehabilitation in Parkinson's?

It might seem that studying exercise or rehabilitation is much easier than studying the effectiveness of new medications. However, studies of exercise have their own challenges. For example, trustworthy drug studies should be "double-blinded" and "placebo-controlled." "Double-blinded" means that both the patient and the investigator are not aware of whether the patient is receiving the study drug. "Placebo-controlled" means that a control group receiving a placebo (so-called sugar pill) is included in the study. In studies of exercise, however, how can you "blind" the study participant? All participants are aware of what types of exercise or rehabilitation they are receiving. The best we can do is to "blind" the investigators who perform the evaluations of the participants; since only one person is blinded, we call this type of study "single-blinding."

We can also perform comparison studies where we compare different types of exercise or rehabilitation training. In this case all study subjects should have a similarly sized placebo effect, so if one study group performs better than another, that is presumably because their exercise training was more effective. Another big challenge in exercise studies is finding enough patients who want to enroll in this type of study. Many people who have Parkinson's are so sedentary that they will not consider enrolling and committing to a vigorous exercise regimen. At the other extreme, the people who tend to be the most enthusiastic about these studies are already engaged in vigorous exercise. This can pose a problem also, since it's more difficult to show the effects of exercise if the study participant has been exercising regularly prior to the start of the study. In addition, studies of exercise training tend to be more time consuming and require a special type of commitment from their participants. In other words, it may be easier to take three tablets a day of study medication and travel to the study site once a month than traveling to the study site three times a week for several months to participate in an exercise trial.

There are many gaps in our knowledge about the effects of exercise and many questions that need to be answered, such as: *What types of exercise are effective in Parkinson's? How much exercise do you need to do to be able to show some benefit? What symptoms respond to exercise? Is exercise beneficial at all stages of Parkinson's? Does exercise slow the progression of Parkinson's?* Many different studies will be necessary to answer these questions. But let's review what we have learned so far.

What Types of Exercise
Are Effective in Parkinson's?

Many types of exercise have been studied in Parkinson's, including treadmill walking, cycling, weight lifting (resistance exercise), swimming, yoga, tai chi, and even dancing and boxing. Reviewing the results of these previous studies demonstrates that many types of exercise are beneficial in Parkinson's. In other words, we are not likely to find that a single type of exercise is the one everyone should do. This makes sense, since people who have Parkinson's have different levels of fitness, different types of symptoms, and different preferences. The majority of studies have focused on training the lower body and trunk ("core muscles"); relatively few studies have investigated exercise training of the arms and hands. In general, this is understandable since the most disabling symptoms of Parkinson's are problems with walking and balance. People who have Parkinson's are generally able to compensate for problems with hand and arm movements (upper body) better than problems with leg movements (lower body). However, we need to increase our knowledge about the effects of exercise on the dexterity of hand movements.

We tend not even to consider cognitive training when we think about exercise training, but it is indeed possible to "exercise the mind" and this is an increasingly active area of study.

A good way to think about the different types of exercise is to divide them into categories. For example, we can consider the following categories: (1) aerobic exercise, (2) muscle strengthening, and (3) stretching (to improve flexibility and range of motion). Another way to categorize exercise is by the region of the body that is the target of the training, such as (1) lower body, (2) upper body, (3) trunk (core), and (4) cognitive training. Yet another approach is to focus on the types of Parkinson's symptoms that you might want to address, such as (1) weakness (poor endurance or deconditioning), (2) walking difficulty, (3) balance problems, (4) loss of hand dexterity, and (5) loss of flexibility (range of motion).

These categories can be a guide to the kinds of exercise that may be right for you. For example, recent evidence has shown that treadmill walking is beneficial for improving both gait speed and aerobic fitness. Weight lifting (resistance exercise) has been shown to improve muscle strength. Studies in seniors who do not have Parkinson's show that people who regularly perform cognitively challenging tasks have less risk for memory difficulties. Combinations of different types of exercise seem to make a lot of sense, but there is very little information about whether the benefits of different types of exercise may be additive or even might have combined effects. So you can think of the different categories described in the previous paragraph as a menu that you use to piece together your own exercise regimen based on your individual needs.

Once you decide to start a specific type of exercise, there are still important decisions to be made about how to get started and how to increase the intensity of exercise over time. For example, if you are starting with treadmill walking to work on your gait and fitness, you will need to make decisions about what settings are best to start with for gait velocity (walking speed) and treadmill incline. The duration of treadmill walking also needs to be decided. Finally, you will need some guidelines about how you will ramp up the intensity of exercise over time. Similarly, if you are beginning resistance exercise to improve your strength, you need to make some early decisions about which regions of the body you want to focus on and what is an appropriate starting weight for you. If you have experience with exercise or if your symptoms are relatively mild, you may be able to get started on your own. If your symptoms are more advanced, if you have been sedentary for a long time, if you have never exercised, or if you have other medical conditions, you will benefit from consultation with a physical therapist or an exercise trainer with experience with Parkinson's and disability. Safety comes first. It's best to start with supervision to prevent injury.

How Much Exercise Do You Need to Do to Show Some Benefit?

Most studies have investigated the effects of performing exercise two to three times per week for thirty to sixty minutes per session. This is a reasonable formula for people who have Parkinson's and for people who do not have Parkinson's. Improvements in performance have been shown within weeks of starting a good exercise regimen. The majority of studies in Parkinson's have assessed the results of two or three months of exercise, but we know from studies of exercise in people who do not have Parkinson's that the benefits continue to mount over much longer periods of time. It's interesting to speculate what the effects of regular physical training over a period of years may have on the different symptoms of Parkinson's. Since the evidence is still lacking, we can hypothesize that it's quite possible that problems with walking, rising from a chair, and general loss of endurance and fatigue may be delayed with regular physical training from the time of diagnosis. A few studies have looked at the effects of stopping rehabilitation therapy or exercise, and these studies show that the benefits of physical training are lost over a period of weeks to months.

WHAT SYMPTOMS RESPOND TO EXERCISE?

It is clear that exercise is beneficial for people who have Parkinson's, but it's important to be realistic about the goals, since some symptoms are more likely to improve than others. Many studies have shown improvements in walking including the speed of walking and endurance. Studies also show improvements of gait rhythm and stride length. It's also clear that cardiovascular fitness improves in people who have Parkinson's following aerobic training such as treadmill walking, cycling, running, or swimming. Muscle strength improves following resistance exercises where the number of repetitions and the resistance weight is gradually increased over time. It is logical to conclude that improvements in walking, fitness, and strength may work in combination to achieve optimum results, although these types of studies still need to be performed.

Not all types of exercise have the same outcomes. Improvements in lower body functions like walking are unlikely to result from upper body training, and muscle strengthening is unlikely to result from treadmill training or cycling. Instead the type of exercise needs to be properly selected to achieve the desired goals. In a recent study where treadmill training and resistance training were compared in people who have

Parkinson's, the people receiving treadmill training improved their cardiovascular fitness but not their muscle strength, and the people receiving resistance training improved their muscle strength but not their fitness. Both the treadmill group and the resistance group showed improvement in the distance they walked over a six-minute period. Since the mechanism of the improvements is different in treadmill vs. resistance exercise, this suggests that combining different types of exercise may have the capacity to achieve even greater benefits.

There is some evidence that exercise may improve balance, but this effect is not as consistently shown in studies, and it is not clear what approach may be best for balance. It seems reasonable that physical training that focuses directly on balance, like tai chi, may be more effective than basic gait training that works on balance more indirectly, but further studies are needed. There is also less consistent evidence that exercise is helpful in improving fatigue or depression. Although many people who exercise report that exercise improves fatigue or depression, some studies show this and some do not. When we consider the cardinal symptoms of Parkinson's (tremor, rigidity, bradykinesia, gait, and balance difficulty), we conclude that exercise training is most likely to be helpful for problems with walking and bradykinesia, may be helpful for rigidity and balance, and is not likely to be helpful for tremor.

Recent evidence suggests that training that is targeted for nonmotor symptoms like cognitive function, speech, and swallowing may be beneficial. Studies are under way to investigate the effects of cognitive training on memory and other cognitive functions. Similar to physical exercise, cognitive training, including computer "games," is targeted for certain types of mental functions, and the difficulty level is gradually ramped up over time. For example, cognitive training may focus on memory, multitasking, attention, or mathematical ability.

Speech therapists use various types of training including an emphasis on increased volume of the voice, particularly using the Lee Silverman Voice Treatment (LSVT) LOUD method (which concentrates on increasing vocal loudness or volume), or exercises focused on pronunciation of sounds to improve problems of soft speech or slurred speech. And there have been recent promising results from studies employing a device that exercises the muscle of the throat that is involved in swallowing (the pharynx) to improve swallowing difficulties. Other nonmotor symptoms like constipation are also improved with increased physical activity.

There is increasing recognition of the importance of performing more than one task simultaneously in daily life. We call this "dual tasking." For example, people generally do not simply walk in isolation, but while walking other tasks are performed simultaneously, including carrying packages, finding your way in an unfamiliar place, and talking on a cell phone. The important part of dual tasking is that you need a combination of motor and cognitive skills to perform these combined tasks. Studies show that both problems with motor function *and* cognitive function interfere with dual tasking. Therefore, it makes sense that exercise training targeted at both motor function (like walking) and cognitive function (multitasking) may improve performance of daily activities. This is significant since problems with dual tasking not only result in difficulties with daily function but also increase the risk of falls. Improving dual-task performance is the focus of ongoing studies.

Of course the main goal is to improve people's daily function and quality of life—to translate these selected improvements to more general improvements in people's daily life and overall well-being. Even though it seems intuitive that improvements in walking, fitness, and strength will result in more pervasive positive effects in the lives of people who have Parkinson's, it can be difficult to demonstrate this outcome in studies. This may be because longer periods of exercise are required or because the effects of exercise are not large enough to achieve this outcome.

Is Exercise Beneficial at All Stages of Parkinson's?

Nearly all of the previous studies of exercise training have enrolled people who have mild to moderate symptoms of Parkinson's. Very few studies have focused on people who have advanced Parkinson's and more complex problems including frequent falls, motor fluctuations, dyskinesia, or significant cognitive dysfunction. Therefore, we have a limited understanding of whether exercise training is beneficial at all stages of Parkinson's. For example, we need more information about what types of exercise are safe and effective at each stage. We are particularly eager to understand whether the progression of Parkinson's might be altered by starting motor and perhaps cognitive training from the time of onset of symptoms and diagnosis.

DOES EXERCISE SLOW
THE PROGRESSION OF PARKINSON'S?

What do we mean by "slowing the progression of Parkinson's"? Some people use this phrase to mean delaying the changes in the brain caused by Parkinson's—in other words, slowing down the loss of brain cells that produce dopamine. Other people use this phrase to mean simply delaying the disability caused by Parkinson's disease without necessarily slowing down the underlying disease process. This difference in meaning is important since it's possible that disability can be delayed without altering the underlying changes in the brain. For example, exercise training might preserve mobility, strength, and endurance, resulting in preserved independent function. Conversely, it's possible that exercise might directly affect the disease process in the brain, but the degree of "neuroprotection" may be too small to result in a clear delay in disability.

In fact, basic science research has shown that exercise *is* neuroprotective in animal models of Parkinson's. Rats and monkeys that are exercised vigorously are protected from the effects of experimental brain injury that causes parkinsonian symptoms. The study animals are generally exercised much more vigorously than human study participants, and ultimately the animals' brain tissue is carefully examined under a microscope. Therefore, the results of animal studies are promising but not definitive. Parkinson's investigators are very eager to study neuroprotection in people who have Parkinson's, but these studies will require large numbers of study participants who will need to be followed for long periods of time—this type of study is labor intensive and expensive. As the evidence continues to mount supporting the benefits of exercise, it is more and more likely that large funding agencies will fund this type of major study.

What Exercise Regimen Is Best for *You*?

There is not one type of exercise regimen that will fit the needs of all people who have Parkinson's. Importantly, current evidence shows that many diverse forms of physical and mental activity are effective and that different types of activity yield different types of benefits. Therefore, combining different types of exercise is the key to a healthy exercise regimen both for people who have Parkinson's disease and for people who don't have Parkinson's disease. The key elements for a physical exercise routine include (1) stretching exercise, (2) aerobic exercise, and (3) resistance exercise. Safety issues are paramount, but it is likely that people at all stages of disease can perform tailored exercise programs. People who have substantial disability can perform stretching exercises, use light weights for muscle strengthening, and train on a recumbent stationary bicycle (cycling while seated with a backrest). People who have moderate disability can perform treadmill training at low speed while holding on to the railings and may be able to use a range of muscle-strengthening machines. People who have early Parkinson's who do not have other active medical conditions are likely to be able to perform a comprehensive exercise routine.

The key elements of success are (1) for each person to start with a realistic view of their level of fitness, strength, and flexibility, (2) training that starts at one's individual level of ability, and (3) gradual ramping up of the level of difficulty over time. Continuing to gradually increase the level of difficulty is important and may be accomplished in many ways. You may increase the duration of your exercise routine by spending more time on the treadmill or bicycle, or you may increase the number of repetitions of your weight lifting or the number and types of stretches you perform. You may increase the intensity of exercise by increasing the amount of weight being lifted or by increasing the velocity or incline on the treadmill. By "pushing the envelope" gradually, at your own individual pace, you will make steady progress and begin to notice the difference in your daily activities. You may notice that by improving the strength of your core muscles (back and abdomen) you can sit up straighter. Or you may feel less winded after walking up a small incline. Or you may find that you lift heavy packages with more ease.

Or that you climb out of the car with less difficulty. Or that you enjoy socializing with family and friends more as your endurance improves. These are meaningful differences in peoples' lives and in fact are similar to the types of results obtained with antiparkinsonian medications. Exercise cannot substitute for medication therapy but is an important supplement to medication therapy. It is clear that the investment you make in exercise will reap meaningful differences in your function over time. As movement disorders specialists we clearly see the differences between our patients who have Parkinson's disease and who remain physically active with routine exercise and those who maintain a sedentary lifestyle—and you will see the difference in yourself, too.

CHAPTER 15

Diet and Complementary/
Alternative Therapies

- *Do special diets help with Parkinson's symptoms?*
- *Do antioxidants protect against Parkinson's?*
- *What kinds of benefits are offered by tai chi or acupuncture?*
- *Why do some physicians discourage patients from using complementary therapies?*

Special diets, vitamin supplements, exercise, rehabilitation, speech therapy, and a host of complementary and alternative therapies—all these approaches to treatment are available in addition to the traditional allopathic (medical) treatments described in Chapters 11, 12, and 13. As physicians, we generally find these approaches acceptable as long as they are not harmful and do not interfere with obtaining proper medical treatment.

Stress reduction techniques are a good example. Meditate. Seek balance in your life. Laugh. Enjoy your grandchildren. Be forthright about your illness so you don't have to put energy into hiding it. Although we don't know whether the therapies described in this chapter enable patients to reduce their medications, many of these therapies do play a role in people's overall well-being and, in that case, are important.

Diet

People who have Parkinson's disease and their families frequently inquire about diet. With a few exceptions described below, no specific dietary therapy is recommended for people who have Parkinson's. A well-balanced diet is important, and people should monitor their weight to be sure it remains stable. Weight gain adds to the stress of moving the body, and weight loss may indicate some other problem and therefore should be reported to the physician. As discussed earlier, patients who have advanced Parkinson's disease often have unexplained weight loss.

If you have Parkinson's, there are no stringent restrictions about what you should eat. Common sense is the best guide. Increasing the amount of fiber in your diet and drinking five to six glasses of water a day will promote healthy bowel habits and help prevent constipation.

If no other health conditions or medications make alcohol consumption inadvisable, people who have Parkinson's may have a glass of wine or beer or a cocktail with their dinner. All the following antiparkinson medications are compatible with the consumption of reasonable amounts of alcohol: immediate-release and controlled-release carbidopa/levodopa (Sinemet and Sinemet CR), selegiline (Eldepryl), and rasagiline (Azilect); all the dopamine receptor agonists—pergolide (Permax), bromocriptine (Parlodel), ropinirole (Requip), pramipexole (Mirapex), and rotigotine patch (Neupro); entacapone (Comtan) and tolcapone (Tasmar); amantadine (Symmetrel); and the anticholinergics—trihexyphenidyl (Artane), benztropine (Cogentin), and procycli dine (Kemadrin). Drugs that are *not* compatible with alcohol include the mild tranquilizers including such examples as diazepam (Valium), alprazolam (Xanax), clorazepate (Tranxene), and lorazepam (Ativan). The atypical antipsychotics quietipine (Seroquel) and clozaril (Clozapine) are also not compatible with alcohol consumption.

Vitamins

First a caveat: in taking any vitamins, but especially for therapeutic purposes, keep in mind that vitamins and minerals are not subject to the rigorous standards of purity and consistency that regulate medicines. Purchasing a reputable brand name from a reputable store may—or may not—help.

There is a hypothesis that vitamin E and vitamin C might protect neurons and delay the degeneration in Parkinson's disease. Both vitamins are *antioxidants*. Oxidation is a chemical reaction that occurs, for example, when iron rusts or when the exposed inside surface of an apple turns brown. When certain molecules in the body are oxidized, damage to the cells can result. If, as one hypothesis suggests, some of the neuron degeneration in Parkinson's is caused by an excess of oxidizing chemicals in the body, taking these oxidizing chemicals out of circulation should help protect the neurons. Antioxidants react with and neutralize the oxidizing chemicals.

From this perspective, we might suppose that antioxidants such as vitamins E and C would help protect the neurons. Vitamin E was put to the test in the DATATOP study, described in Chapter 13. Vitamin E failed the test, however, even though study participants were given 2,000 units a day. Higher doses might be beneficial, but the side effects could also be serious. In fact, recent publications suggest that vitamin E in higher doses may be harmful.

The next question is whether vitamin C may offer neuroprotection, at levels of 2 to 3 grams a day. The studies of vitamin C use by Parkinson's patients have been small and the results inconclusive: we cannot conclude that vitamin C has any neuroprotective role.

Another antioxidant that has been tried in well-organized, controlled clinical research trials supported by the NIH is high-dose Coenzyme Q_{10} (CoQ_{10}). In dosages as high as 2,400 mg/day, CoQ_{10} did not slow progression of Parkinson's in patients with early untreated disease. Although disappointing, it is important for the patient community to know about this failure, since many patients were spending considerable amounts of money to purchase CoQ_{10} with the hope that the trial would be positive.

Other vitamins are of interest, too. Vitamin B_6 (pyridoxine) has been a source of confusion for many people because of work published decades ago. Vitamin B_6 has many functions in the body, one of which is to boost the enzyme that converts levodopa to dopamine. In the late 1960s and early 1970s, when levodopa alone was used to treat Parkinson's disease (before the introduction of carbidopa/levodopa), some researchers hypothesized that giving vitamin B$_6$ in conjunction with levodopa might help relieve symptoms of Parkinson's. The idea was that adding vitamin B$_6$ to the diet could enhance the enzymatic process, increasing the rate of conversion of levodopa to dopamine.

In practice, when people took vitamin B$_6$ and *levodopa alone*, the reverse happened—the Parkinson's symptoms worsened. This occurred because vitamin B$_6$ boosts the conversion of levodopa to dopamine both within and outside the brain. More vitamin B$_6$ converted more levodopa outside the brain to dopamine. Dopamine, as you will recall, cannot cross the blood-brain barrier into the brain, and thus the brain's motor control system was not helped by increased dopamine in the blood. Given the worsening of symptoms, people who have Parkinson's were advised to avoid vitamin B$_6$ while taking levodopa.

When carbidopa/levodopa (Sinemet) was introduced, the story changed. Because the enzyme that converts levodopa to dopamine is blocked by carbidopa, vitamin B$_6$ is no longer a problem. Levodopa is rarely used alone today, and vitamin B$_6$ is compatible with Sinemet (carbidopa/levodopa), Sinemet CR, or the benserazide/levodopa preparations (Prolopa, Madopar) available outside the United States. Multivitamin tablets with 5 to 10 milligrams of vitamin B$_6$ and breakfast cereals fortified with vitamin B$_6$ do not pose any problems. Finally, you may hear about the use of intravenous (IV) administration of gluatathione (another antioxidant) for Parkinson's disease. There is little evidence that this treatment provides significant benefit, and this is not an accepted therapy for Parkinson's disease.

Protein Redistribution Diet

A few people who have Parkinson's who are taking levodopa do need to follow a special diet—the protein redistribution diet, described in detail in Chapter 13. The diet simply shifts the time when a person eats protein from early to late in the day.

To summarize: after a meal heavy in protein, some people taking levodopa find they have trouble with motor fluctuations or other signs that their levodopa isn't functioning well. This occurs because amino acids from the protein in food compete with levodopa (also an amino acid) for the pathways from the small intestine to the bloodstream, and then from the bloodstream into the brain. Thus less of the levodopa dose actually reaches the brain, and the dose of drug a person has taken is less effective than it should be. One solution is for people who notice such a reaction to eat their protein in the evening, when mobility isn't as important, rather than during the day. Although the timing of protein consumption changes in this diet, people still need to get enough protein to avoid other health problems.

As emphasized in Chapter 13, this diet is useful only for people who are taking levodopa and have noticed increased motor fluctuations when they consume meals high in protein. The diet is not helpful to people who have early Parkinson's who are not on medication or for people taking only dopamine receptor agonists, MAO inhibitors, anticholinergics, or amantadine, none of which compete for the same pathways in the way that protein and levodopa do.

Alternative Dietary Supplements

A host of dietary supplements are marketed as potential therapeutic agents for people who have Parkinson's disease. These include over-the-counter antioxidants, food supplements, ginkgo biloba, ginseng, herbal preparations, massive doses of vitamins, Coenzyme Q_{10} (CoQ_{10}), and NADH preparations (a supplement reputed to help Parkinson's disease). None of these supplements has been proven to be of value in treating Parkinson's disease, nor have we ever observed any useful therapeutic effect from them. These items are not regulated and have varying degrees of purity.

COMPLEMENTARY AND ALTERNATIVE MEDICINE

People may seek alternatives to traditional allopathic medical approaches. Our patients with Parkinson's disease employ a wide range of alternative therapies. These include acupuncture, chelation therapy, and spa treatments.

The routine variations in Parkinson's symptoms from day to day make it difficult to judge whether alternative therapies are effective in the long term or may be useful for brief periods. The development of traditional treatments involved years of intensive research, and this kind of research has not yet been done for alternative therapies.

For example, acupuncture needs to be subjected to the same scrutiny we apply to all therapies, in accordance with sound scientific principles. Very few, if any, reports in the lay press on nontraditional therapies such as acupuncture are based on controlled clinical trials. Chinese medicine is based on premises quite different from those of Western medicine, and research on these is only just beginning. We need clear-cut answers about the role of alternative therapies in the treatment of Parkinson's disease before recommending any of them.

Acupuncture

Acupuncture is the use of needles to balance the body's energy, known as *chi*. According to Chinese medical studies, chi flows along body lines called *meridians*, which you may have seen displayed on Chinese acupuncture charts. The acupuncturist determines where flow may be blocked or may be moving too rapidly, then places needles in accordance with the assessment.

Acupuncture has been most successfully applied for pain syndromes and problems of addiction and substance abuse. Currently, there is little or no data to suggest that standard and especially the highly touted "ear-implant" acupunture is effective for relieving the symptoms of Parkinson's disease, and no evidence that it in any way slows down the progress of Parkinson's. One study of acupuncture in Parkinson's showed some improvement of sleep habits but no change of any of the main symptoms of the disease.

Acupuncture may help people feel more in balance with their lives and perhaps generally healthier. Some people who have Parkinson's who receive acupuncture find it relaxing or find their various aches and pains are relieved. As long as acupuncture is used in conjunction with a doctor's recommendations, it probably does no harm and might be useful.

Chelation Therapy

Chelation therapy is another nontraditional approach used by people seeking alternative treatment. Chelation therapy is the intravenous administration of chelating agents, which remove metals and some other substances from the body. Chelating agents are used in traditional Western medicine to treat intoxications or overdoses with certain metals, such as lead. But there is no evidence that metal exposure is associated with Parkinson's disease and thus no rational basis for chelation therapy in Parkinson's disease.

Those who practice chelation therapy suggest that the chelating agent also removes other "poisons" present in the body that might contribute to Parkinson's disease. Again, these claims have no reasonable theoretical basis.

In addition, chelation therapy poses some dangers. First, chelating agents are not very specific about what they remove from the body, and they can pull out necessary metals and minerals such as iron and calcium. Because the treatments may involve intravenous injections, they pose a risk of infection and development of blood clots that can block essential blood vessels.

Chelation therapy for Parkinson's disease is not covered by Medicare or other government insurance plans, nor is it covered by most major insurance carriers. Despite the absence of any proof that this therapy works, and despite the risks associated with the use of chelating agents, some patients and families pay large sums of money to receive chelation therapy. In our view, however, chelation therapy currently has no role in the treatment of Parkinson's.

Spa Treatments

There are spas, and then there are spas. Many people who have Parkinson's disease show their doctors advertisements touting help or even cures for their Parkinson's at a spa, often in Germany, Switzerland, or Eastern Europe. The problems with these spas lie in their extravagant claims and in the therapies they offer. Therapies include special diets, various forms of baths, massage, injection of chelating agents, and injection of fetal cells from sheep or cows.

The fetal cell therapy is based on the idea that injecting the embryonic cells of sheep or cows will cause the body to rejuvenate (not the same as fetal transplantation, discussed in Chapter 16). This has never been demonstrated to be of value in treating any disorder, including Parkinson's disease. Moreover, injection of anything into the body carries some risks of local abscesses or infection.

A stay at a European health spa may cost from $10,000 to $15,000 for seven to fourteen days in Switzerland and Germany, or $5,000 to $10,000 for similar amounts of time in Poland, Hungary, or Romania. Spending this amount of money for a relaxing vacation, if you can comfortably afford to do so, is one thing. But spending this money if you cannot afford it or spending the money in search of a promised help or cure that will not help, will not cure, and may even do harm is something else altogether.

Why Are Physicians Concerned about Alternative Therapies?

As physicians who see many patients with Parkinson's disease, we understand there are times when they and their families feel hopeless, times when they feel desperate about their medical situation. In those moments, they may turn to alternative therapies, no matter how unrealistic or far-fetched they appear or how much they cost.

A physician's role is to be a trusted resource for patients and their families. The doctor has current information on the range of therapies: which are dangerous; which are uncertain; which might feel good and change little else; which are unproven, but may eventually prove useful; and which are proven, effective therapies. Thus, when a patient arrives at the physician's office enthusiastic about a new treatment, the physician may seem unnecessarily skeptical or overly critical of this alternative therapy. This skepticism, however, reflects a physician's store of information as well as years of education and training, which stress that medical recommendations need to be based on scientific data, not just on opinion or intuition. Fortunately, funding is increasingly available from the National Institutes of Health to study complementary and alternative therapies.

Just because a treatment makes logical or emotional sense does not mean that it works. Again, a therapy that increases someone's comfort without endangering him or her in any way is probably a good thing. But, to paraphrase, *first it should do no harm.*

CHAPTER 16

Surgical Treatments

- *What are the risks of neurosurgery, and what are the benefits?*
- *Which surgical procedures have been accepted and practiced by doctors, and which procedures are still being developed?*
- *What tools can a patient use to evaluate the skill and expertise of a neurosurgeon?*
- *What factors determine whether surgery is right for a particular individual?*

For decades, neurosurgeons have investigated the connection between the anatomy of the brain and the symptoms of Parkinson's disease. By interrupting various neural circuits within the brain, accomplished by carefully destroying a region of brain tissue in order to create a *lesion,* surgeons have sought to reduce a person's symptoms of tremor, rigidity, slowness, and postural problems. Neurosurgeons did not expect these procedures to cure or even delay progression of the disease, but they hoped to improve the symptoms and quality of life in people who have advanced Parkinson's for whom medications were no longer as effective as they had been.

In Chapter 11 we discussed how the signal for movement originates in the brain cortex and travels through multiple concentric loops within the brain for feedback and modulation, before eventually passing to a muscle. When Parkinson's disrupts the substantia nigra–dopamine system, the groups of neurons "downstream" from the disruption sometimes become hyperactive, and this causes some of the Parkinson's symptoms. A surgically produced lesion destroys some of this abnormal hyperactivity by restoring the balance of signals, and thus relieves the symptoms.

Although creating a brain lesion may help alleviate the symptoms of Parkinson's, surgery does not cure or even slow the disease. Parkinson's remains a degenerative disease: it continues to get worse. Some neurosurgical centers report that some of the benefits of the surgery last for more than five years. Other centers report that some of the benefits begin to disappear after about a year. People who have Parkinson's might ask, "If I have this surgery and it's useful to me for two years, is that worth it?" For some people, the answer is yes.

Surgical treatments for Parkinson's disease began in the 1930s, before the development of levodopa, and produced notably uneven results. Surgical lesions were mostly aimed at reducing tremor, but they also created new neurologic deficits such as paralysis and slurred speech. By the end of the 1960s, surgical strategies had evolved and neurosurgeons had learned which areas of the brain responded best to surgery and which surgical "targets" produced the fewest side effects. Thereafter, surgery focused on two brain structures: the *thalamus* and the *globus pallidus*. The thalamus contains a number of distinct cell groups that are involved in complex relays—some of them from the globus pallidus—in the motor control circuits discussed in Chapter 11. Physicians thought *thalamotomy* (the selective destruction of a small portion of the thalamus) and *pallidotomy* (the selective destruction of a small area of the globus pallidus) both offered potential relief from parkinsonian tremor and rigidity.

These neurosurgical procedures were in use in the 1950s and 1960s, before the levodopa era. Yet even then, the use of this "functional" neurosurgery (meaning surgery intended to improve *functioning*, not provide a cure) was not widespread. Such procedures provided benefits too inconsistently, and too frequently produced adverse effects. Surgery was used as a treatment for severe tremor, however, because very few useful medications were available.

Levodopa, highly effective in alleviating Parkinson's symptoms, emerged in the late 1960s, and many neurologists and neurosurgeons lost their enthusiasm for the surgical procedures with their attendant risks. The use of thalamotomy and pallidotomy virtually ceased, except in a few countries, including Sweden and Japan. Interest in thalamotomy has never been revived in the United States, because levodopa continues to be effective for treating the same symptoms relieved by this procedure and thalamotomy is effective only for tremor relief.

Pallidotomy has seen something of a resurgence in North America. The procedure resurfaced in the 1990s, in part because neurosurgeons have been able to make significant improvements in their techniques and now better understand the neural circuits that give rise to Parkinson's symptoms. In addition, drug-induced dyskinesia—which in the 1960s, before levodopa was available, did not exist—is now a more common problem, one that responds well to surgical treatment. On the other hand, lesioning techniques, including pallidotomy, have been largely supplanted by the use of deep brain stimulation of various targets, particularly the subthalamic nucleus but also the globus pallidus and, to a lesser extent, the thalamus.

Our discussion of neurosurgical approaches to Parkinson's disease focuses on five different procedures:

1. Thalamotomy and pallidotomy, the placement of lesions in the thalamus or globus pallidus
2. Deep brain stimulation of the thalamus, globus pallidus, or subthalamic nucleus
3. Nerve cell transplantation
4. Injection of nerve cell growth factors into the brain
5. Injection of various gene vectors into the brain

The first two of these approaches are currently in use, whereas nerve cell transplantation and injection of nerve cell growth factors and gene vectors are available only through research programs that are investigating their safety and effectiveness.

Undergoing a surgical procedure is quite different from taking a drug. The risks from neurosurgery are significant, including stroke, brain hemorrhage (rarely resulting in death), slurred speech, postoperative confusion, changes in thinking and behavior, and infection at the site of the hole in the skull or even in the brain. Patients should be sure that if they choose to have surgery, the surgery is performed at a surgical center that has extensive experience with that particular procedure.

Reputable centers will inform the prospective patient about how many surgical procedures have been performed, how many people got better, which symptoms improved, and the frequency and type of complications that resulted from the operation. These centers generally are located at a major medical center and have a team of neurologists, neurosurgeons, electrophysiologists, neuropsychologists, neuropsychiatrists, and nurses with considerable expertise in the evaluation and management of Parkinson's. Individuals considering surgery need to fully evaluate the potential risks and benefits of the surgical option and put this option into perspective with other available therapies.

Although some of these surgical procedures are already in use to treat Parkinson's symptoms, continued research is needed to adequately define the specific population of people who have Parkinson's who will benefit from each procedure. The currently available operations generally do not improve symptoms that have been unresponsive to levodopa, with the exception of tremor. Specifically, surgery will generally not improve the freezing and falling that occur even during "on" times, nor will it improve speech function. Thinking and memory problems may worsen after surgery, sometimes considerably.

In short, none of these procedures is without significant risk. At the end of this chapter we provide an important list of questions you should ask yourself, your doctor, and the surgeon when considering whether to undergo any brain surgery for Parkinson's disease.

THALAMOTOMY AND PALLIDOTOMY

Before performing thalamotomy or pallidotomy, surgeons and movement disorder specialists identify the target region of the brain by using one of several methods, including special computerized imaging systems, electrophysiologic recording from neurons in the brain, and special anatomic atlases. They also identify the nearby structures to avoid when creating the lesion.

During the surgery, a hole is made in the skull and thin probes with electrodes are passed through the hole to the target region. The patient is awake during the surgery. The patient does not experience pain but can have considerable discomfort associated with remaining on the operative table for a long period. During the procedure, the surgeon or the neurologist asks the patient to perform repetitive movements, such as opening and closing the hand and speaking, to confirm that the probe is located accurately in the target. Patients are frequently aware of the moment when their tremor or rigidity improves during the surgical procedure.

After the precise brain site has been identified, the surgeon gradually heats up the tip of the electrode until it irreversibly injures a small amount of brain tissue in the target area. In a thalamotomy, a small region in the thalamus is destroyed. This procedure is primarily useful for people who have severe tremor; it may also relieve rigidity. Thalamotomy does little or nothing for other disabling features of Parkinson's such as slowness, clumsiness of movement, or walking difficulties and, as noted above, it is now seldom performed.

In a pallidotomy, a small region in the globus pallidus is destroyed. The current pallidotomy procedure creates a lesion in a slightly different area of the globus pallidus than did the older procedure. A lesion created in this new target area reliably affects Parkinson's symptoms. Many Parkinson's centers have now reported that this procedure is especially beneficial for drug-induced dyskinesia and can also relieve tremor, rigidity, and bradykinesia.

Because pallidotomy using the previous, somewhat different target had already been recognized as a standard neurosurgical procedure, surgeons have been able to resume performing the procedure without extensive clinical trials. Surgical procedures are not held to the same standard as pharmaceuticals. In North America, before a drug is made available to the public for specific purposes, extensive testing must be done to demonstrate that it is both safe and effective. The same is not true of surgical procedures that have previously been in use.

In our view, pallidotomy should not be undertaken lightly. One reason is the continuing debate in the neurologic community about its proper role in treating Parkinson's disease. Some neurologists believe pallidotomy is appropriate mainly for people experiencing severe drug-induced dyskinesia. Other neurologists believe pallidotomy should be used for people who have advanced Parkinson's who are having increasing difficulty with basic symptoms of the disease such as tremor, slowness, stiffness, and walking. However, the number of pallidotomies has decreased in recent years, because physicians' and patients' interest has shifted to the use of deep brain stimulation.

ADVANTAGES OF LESIONING techniques over deep brain stimulation (described below) are the following: usually, there is only need for a single surgery; no foreign materials (electrodes) are implanted; there is no need for a second operation to implant the power source on the chest wall; there is less risk of recurrent infection; and there are no hardware or software issues postoperatively and no need for frequent DBS programming visits. As emphasized below, the downsides relate to the possible permanent nature of complications of a lesion, the inability to titrate the treatment according to response (as in DBS programming), and the poor safety of lesion surgery involving both sides of the brain ("bilateral") in contrast to the much safer use of bilateral DBS.

Another method of lesioning the thalamus or the pallidus without an open operation is the use of focused radiation with a *gamma knife*. Proponents of this technique argue that it is noninvasive and safer, especially for frail elderly patients or for patients in whom standard functional surgery is contraindicted (e.g., those with bleeding tendencies or who are taking anticoagulants). However, most functional neurosurgeons feel that this technique has problems, including the accuracy necessary to obtain optimal benefit, and side effects, due to the spread of the radiation-induced lesion beyond the desired area. A very recently developed technique for lesioning the brain in a noninvasive way is with focused ultrasound. Unlike the gamma knife, results are seen immediately, and lesioning (heating) can be stopped before major permanent side effects develop. This tool remains experimental for brain lesioning, and it is not clear what role it will play in the treatment of Parkinson's in the future.

DEEP BRAIN STIMULATION

An important and now well-established surgical approach, deep brain stimulation (DBS) operates on a principle similar to pallidotomy or thalamotomy, except that in DBS a small area of the brain is *electrically stimulated* rather than destroyed. A neurosurgeon uses a probe to precisely place a small electrode at a specific location in the brain so as to interfere with the functioning of that area. Exactly how DBS works is still not completely understood. Initially, scientists believed that the electrical stimulation caused a temporary blockade of function in that area of the brain. We now know that the effects are probably more complex than this and could even vary depending on the site in the brain that is stimulated.

If DBS has an undesirable outcome, as long as the problem relates to the stimulation and not to complications of the implantation surgery itself, the stimulating electrodes can simply be turned off or the strength of the stimulus can be adjusted. This is very different from the situation with thalamotomy and pallidotomy, both of which are irreversible. If a surgically created lesion leads to a bad outcome, such as a disturbance in the person's vision, there is no way to reverse the process. This is particularly risky in surgery performed on both sides of the brain, and these bilateral lesions result in a relatively high incidence of permanent complications, especially speech disturbances. Because of its reversibility, DBS should carry a lower risk, especially when applied to both sides of the brain.

In the DBS procedure, the Parkinson's team targets the area of the brain where they want to interfere with the functioning of brain circuits, make a hole in the skull, and insert the probe in a process very similar to thalamotomy and pallidotomy. Again, the patient is awake in order to provide feedback to the team for the electrode placement. When the team is satisfied with the placement, the final stimulating electrode is put in place.

A second procedure then follows, either immediately or up to a week later. With the patient under general anesthesia, the surgeon connects the electrode to a wire that runs under the skin to a stimulating box placed in a pouch under the skin on the chest wall. The box and the wire provide the electrical stimulus for the electrode. The arrangement is very similar to the placement of the power source of a cardiac pacemaker (Figure 16.1). Thus, in contrast to pallidotomy or thalamotomy, DBS requires two surgical procedures, one under general anesthetic.

Once the "pacemaker" is implanted, the patient can easily turn the stimulation on or off. When the stimulation is turned on, an electrical current passes from the electrode to the target region and temporarily disrupts the function of that area of the brain.

Deep brain stimulation has been approved for use in the United States and Canada for the treatment of Parkinson's. The target area can be the thalamus, globus pallidus, or subthalamic nucleus (STN). DBS of the thalamus is performed infrequently in Parkinson's since its effect is primarily limited to tremor reduction, whereas DBS of the

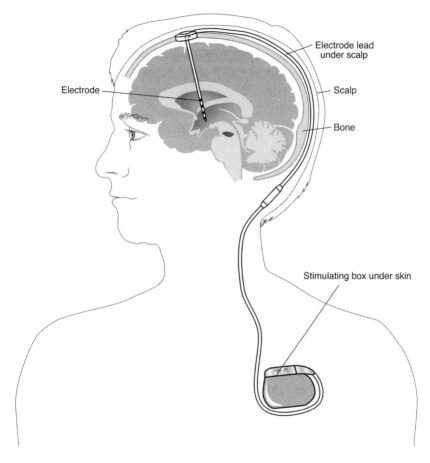

FIGURE 16.1 This figure illustrates the placement of the deep-brain stimulating electrode in the areas of the brain that are involved in motor dysfunction in Parkinson's disease. The techniques for deep brain stimulation involve the placement of the electrode in this region deep within the brain, with the top portion being just beneath the scalp and the wire running beneath the skin of the chest wall to its stimulating box (similar to the situation with a cardiac pacemaker). This figure shows only one side of the brain connected and stimulated. Most patients receiving subthalamic nucleus or globus pallidus stimulation undergo operations on both sides of the brain, and the two electrodes are connected to a single pulse generator (stimulating box).

globus pallidus and STN effectively relieves other disabling symptoms of Parkinson's disease as well as tremor.

If you are considering DBS for the tremor associated with Parkinson's disease, remember that tremor is a very common symptom in Parkinson's disease, which often responds very well to antiparkinson medications, although the dose of levodopa sometimes needed is quite a bit higher than for other symptoms (and may be more than many physicians are used to using). Also, tremor usually decreases when a patient makes a purposeful movement and therefore may not cause much functional disability. The only people for whom DBS placement for tremor should be considered are those with severe, incapacitating tremor that is unresponsive to medications. Those with mild or moderate tremor should not undergo the risk of DBS placement in the thalamus. When tremor is the sole or major reason for surgery, some centers first give a trial of clozapine, the atypical antipsychotic discussed in Chapter 13. Clozapine can have a considerable antitremor effect and in some patients may make it unnecessary to consider surgery.

Recent years have seen a dramatic increase in the number of DBS procedures being performed for treatment of Parkinson's. Most of these procedures target the subthalamic nucleus (STN) and not the globus pallidus (GPi). Although there is no definitive evidence to prove that the STN is a better target than the GPi, clinical practice has certainly moved almost exclusively to deep brain stimulation of the STN to alleviate the motor symptoms of Parkinson's disease. A recent study involving the U.S. Veteran's Administration has raised further questions about the superiority of STN over GPi deep brain stimulation and, like previous studies, it found a slightly higher rate of adverse effects from STN stimulation. However, this study did not obtain the degree of benefit with either target reported in previous studies of STN stimulation, so the results are somewhat hard to interpret. In addition, follow-up was relatively short, and some past studies have suggested that GPi stimulation could become less effective with time and that some patients losing benefit of GPi stimulation received STN stimulation with recovery of benefit. Certainly more data are required before this important issue is resolved.

Deep brain stimulation of the STN has proved very effective in alleviating not only tremors but rigidity and slowness. It is also effective in alleviating dyskinesia, although this effect is probably more related to most people being able to reduce their antiparkinson medications after DBS placement (whereas GPi stimulation seems to have more antidyskinesia effects distinct from the reduction of antiparkinson medications). Significantly, for many people who have DBS performed on both sides of the brain, "off" time is reduced and, on average, they have as much as six additional hours of "on" time. It is important to understand that DBS is not capable of improving a person's best "on" response to levodopa aside from reducing the additional problems caused by dyskinesia. This understanding is critical in selecting individuals for surgery. This surgery is not appropriate for those who have substantial disability even in the best "on" state (e.g., slowness, walking problems, freezing, falling, severe speech problems).

At some movement disorder centers, the electrodes are placed on both sides of the brain during a single operation, and at other centers, the electrode placement is accomplished in two separate procedures. There are advantages to both methods.

Deep brain stimulation of the STN has become a useful treatment for people who have moderate to advanced Parkinson's. It is not a cure. It is also not for everyone with Parkinson's. In choosing a movement disorder center for possible DBS treatment, you need to consider the entire team of specialists who will be taking care of you during the procedure. The team consists of a movement disorder neurologist, neurosurgeon, electrophysiologist (the doctor who reads the electrical activity of the brain during surgery), neuropsychiatrist, neuropsychologist, and nursing staff.

Only people who have Parkinson's who may benefit from this surgery should be selected for the procedure. This seems almost silly to say, but there is no benefit in placing electrodes in the brain unless there is a good chance that it will help. People who have Parkinson's must understand that this procedure is no cure. You and your family should not have unrealistic expectations for the surgery (this is usually determined by a neuropsychiatrist), and it is important that complete agreement be reached between you and the surgical team on the clear goals and expectations of surgery. It is also essential that the diagnosis of Parkinson's is correct (as determined by your movement disorder specialist), that you have no unsuspected cognitive or thinking problems (as determined by special neuropsychological testing), that you are getting a good response to levodopa (as determined by examination

TABLE 16.1

IMPORTANT CONSIDERATIONS IN DBS SURGERY

Correct diagnosis
Continued good response to levodopa
No unrealistic expectations about the surgery
No hidden cognitive or thinking problems
Good general health

in both the "on" and "off" states), and that the neurosurgeon agrees that you are a suitable person for the procedure (see Table 16.1).

The surgical placement of the DBS electrode is accompanied by the same risks associated with other brain surgery: brain hemorrhage, stroke, partial loss of vision, infection, and paralysis. Because DBS requires the long-term placement of an electrode in the brain, connected by wires to a stimulator box in the upper chest, there are additional possibilities for complications, including infection at these remote sites or mechanical breakdowns that may require additional surgical corrections.

In the postoperative period, DBS requires repeated assessments to make sure the stimulation parameters and antiparkinson drugs are optimal for the individual. These assessments can be time consuming and require considerable expertise to obtain the best clinical response with minimum side effects. In the initial days to weeks, patients may experience a variety of symptoms that could be the effects of excessive stimulation or stimulation at less than optimal sites, or of the need to adjust antiparkinson medications—either increase doses toward preoperative levels (if they have been reduced too quickly) or reduce doses, depending on the symptoms experienced. Therefore, close contact with and regular assessments by the neurologic team are essential during this early "programming" period.

Surgeons are regularly considering new targets for stimulation that might be effective in improving symptoms that are relatively resistant to current surgical techniques. As we have emphasized, STN and GPi DBS are not effective for freezing and falling that persist despite optimal levodopa therapy. The pedunculopontine nucleus (PPN) is another region in the brain, located just below the STN, which is probably involved in normal ambulation and postural stability. A limited number of studies have evaluated the use of PPN stimulation in Parkinson's disease, and the results are conflicting. What is clear is that this PPN treatment is not the "answer" that was hoped for these problems. Further research is clearly required. We would recommend considering PPN stimulation treatment only in the context of a research protocol conducted by a well-established academic surgical program.

NERVE CELL TRANSPLANTATION

Another area of particular interest in surgical approaches to treating Parkinson's disease is nerve cell transplantation. The history of nerve cell transplantation began in the 1980s, when there was interest in transplanting *adrenal gland cells*, not nerve cells, into the brain of a person who has Parkinson's. The tale of adrenal cell transplantation is a cautionary one. The principle behind the procedure was that cells could be taken from the adrenal gland in a patient's abdomen and inserted into her or his brain, where they would convert to dopamine-producing cells. At first the procedure was favorably reported in the medical literature, and the public media also covered the story. A considerable number of people underwent the transplantation, even though it was quite a major surgical procedure involving both abdominal surgery to remove the cells from the adrenal gland and neurosurgery to implant the cells into the brain. Subsequently, adrenal cell transplantation was found to be ineffective, and a review of the initial reports revealed that the early enthusiasm was based on highly suspect evidence. Adrenal cell transplantation into the brain has now been abandoned.

The principle behind transplanting nerve cells into the brain is similar. Interest has been focused on human fetal cell transplantation. *Human fetal cell transplantation* is an experimental procedure. Nerve cells destined to become substantia nigra cells are taken from the brains of several aborted human fetuses in early development then implanted into the brain of the person who has Parkinson's disease in the area where dopamine receptors are located. (Recall that the substantia nigra is the area that degenerates in Parkinson's.) The hope is that the human fetal cells will branch out, make contact with the dopamine receptors, and restore the motor control function.

Researchers in Sweden have been interested in this procedure for more than two decades. Over many years, Swedish centers have been following up on a small group of people who have undergone this procedure and have reported symptomatic improvement. Nonetheless, the Swedes concur that the procedure remains experimental. Several other countries, including Cuba and China, have centers where human fetal cell transplantation is available. Well-documented reports of patients who have undergone the transplantation procedures in these countries have not been presented in the scientific literature, so we can draw no conclusions.

Despite the enormous favorable publicity about fetal cell transplantation for Parkinson's, two well-conducted clinical trials sponsored by the National Institutes of Health have investigated whether or not fetal cell transplants actually have any benefit in Parkinson's. The first trial consisted of one group of Parkinson's patients receiving fetal cell implantations and a second group receiving "sham" surgery (surgery that "goes through the motions" but does not actually implant any cells; the sham surgery is thus a type of placebo). Sometime after the surgery, the investigators asked the study participants to answer questions about how well their symptoms were responding. Little difference in symptoms was reported by the two groups and, in people over the age of sixty, no difference was reported at all. The second trial compared a sham surgery group with groups that received transplanted cells from one to four fetuses per side of the brain. Once again, this study failed to show benefit from the fetal transplantation. Importantly, some of the patients in both of these studies developed disabling dyskinesia as a complication of the transplantation, which unlike drug-related dyskinesia, has persisted despite withdrawal of dopaminergic drugs. The development of so-called runaway dyskinesia has markedly slowed clinical trials exploring this idea. It is generally agreed in the research community that this unusual adverse event needs to be better understood before further large trials are conducted. This is particularly important because, overall, little motor benefit was observed. Even if these trials had been successful, it seems unlikely that this therapy will become widely used. The procedure requires an extensive team of investigators to harvest the fetal cells, test the cells for infection, store the cells, dissect the cells, and finally, transplant them into the patient's brain. This procedure involves enormous time and effort, requires a large number of fetuses (up to eight per patient), and poses a number of serious ethical issues. However, based on the considerable benefit experienced by some patients undergoing fetal transplantation and the apparent relationship between transplant-induced dyskinesias and preexisting levodopa-induced dykinesias, a new transplant research program has been developed (largely based in England and Europe but also involving researchers in Canada and the United States) with the plan to study newer transplant techniques in patients at earlier stages of the disease. Finally, we should mention the important recent finding that some patients who survived for ten or more years after fetal transplantation and died from unrelated problems were found to have Lewy bodies (the microscopic brain inclusion of Parkinson's disease) not only in their own brain cells (as expected) but also in the transplanted fetal cells. This suggests that the pathological hallmark feature can somehow be transmitted to other cells placed in the "environment" of the Parkinson's brain. The relevance of this finding to transplantation treatment is uncertain (since it occurred many years after the treatment and may not have influenced the function of the cells to that time), but it has raised some intriguing ideas about how Parkinson's disease normally progresses to involve different regions of the brain over many years.

Considerable attention has been devoted to finding a substitute for human fetal cells. The transplantation of porcine (pig) cells was discussed thoroughly in the last edition of this book as a promising therapy. Porcine cell transplantation has now been abandoned, since it did not work. We mention it here again only to point out that many therapies when first introduced are widely praised and touted, but with time and careful examination, unfortunately, most fail. The tale of the porcine transplants reminds us again how difficult it is to find real and promising therapies.

NERVE GROWTH FACTORS AND "GENE THERAPIES"

Another therapy that has been investigated is the use of nerve growth factors, which may provide new approaches to treatment. Nerve growth factors (also called *neurotrophic factors*) are chemical substances within the brain that facilitate the survival and development of nerve cells. We have discussed in earlier chapters how nerve cells use chemicals called neurotransmitters (such as dopamine) to communicate with one another. Neurotrophic factors are additional chemicals within the brain that are critical for nerve cell survival.

Of the several different types of neurotrophic factors identified, *glial-derived neurotrophic factor* (GDNF) is one of the most important to the survival and growth of dopamine-producing cells. Some researchers suggest that GDNF can improve survival of the dopamine-producing nerve cells in people who have Parkinson's, improve their symptoms, and perhaps even slow down the progress of Parkinson's. GDNF has been shown to work well in monkeys. Unfortunately, this is another example of a potential therapy that seems to work very well in animals but so far not in people who have Parkinson's.

GDNF is a very large molecule and cannot cross the blood-brain barrier, so it cannot be taken by mouth or by the usual injection techniques. Delivery of GDNF to the brain requires surgery. There have been two different approaches to delivery of GDNF to the brain of people who have Parkinson's. In the first trial of GDNF, the chemical was delivered into the ventricles (the large fluid-filled spaces in every brain) via a special catheter (very narrow tube) passing through a small hole in the skull. This trial failed, and many researchers believed that GDNF failed to improve Parkinson's symptoms because it entered the fluid-filled space and never really got to the site in the brain where it was needed. A second trial of GDNF delivered the chemical directly into brain tissue ("intraparenchymal" injection) in the region most affected by dopamine deficiency in Parkinson's (the putamen) via another type of catheter. This trial was stopped for several reasons: there was no statistically significant beneficial effect, some patients developed antibodies to GDNF, and some reports suggested that GDNF might produce abnormalities in the brain of certain animals.

There was considerable publicity associated with the decision to stop the trial, because some people who had received the drug felt they had benefited. But overall, there was no evidence that intraparenchymal injection of GDNF helped in Parkinson's disease. This is another example of why it is so important to conduct rigorous clinical research trials. It would be a sad outcome indeed if, on the basis of an isolated beneficial response in a single person, we started injecting GDNF into thousands of people who have Parkinson's and then found out that it didn't work or, worse, that it caused harm.

GDNF remains a very interesting substance that may yet find a role in the therapy of Parkinson's. Researchers who have treated a small number of patients with different doses of GDNF and using differ- ent types of catheters than were used in the placebo-controlled trial described above continue to argue that their patients have benefited from the treatment and further experimental studies with GDNF con- tinue. Some researchers are now working on delivering genes into the brain that will produce excess GDNF or related growth factors as a way of treating Parkinson's. Gene therapy using a GDNF-related trophic factor, neurturin, initially showed promising but inconclusive findings; however, a more recent study failed to show significant benefit.

IN FACT several reported surgical trials of inserting gene therapies into various brain sites in Parkinson's disease herald the dawn of new re- search endeavors. There is great research interest in gene therapy for Parkinson's disease, and we are now just at the beginning of rudi- mentary attempts to treat Parkinson's disease by inserting "corrective" genes. The idea in all of these trials is to insert a gene that makes a product that enhances dopamine activity or alters a circuit in the brain that is believed to be involved in the symptomatology of Parkinson's disease. The idea is that the corrective gene will enter the brain, enter the nerve cells, produce its product normally and relieve Parkinson's disease symptoms. The genes are delivered to the brain sites by a tech- nique very similar to what we described for the implantation of DBS electrodes, except that when the special tubes are in place, the gene vector is injected and all the hardware is withdrawn. The gene vector is the carrier for the corrective gene. It is a specially altered virus that can infect the brain cells and deliver the gene. The virus has been altered so that it is no longer capable of causing any brain infections or damage to the cells that receive the virus. The initial results of this type of gene therapy have shown moderate results in terms of altering symptoms of Parkinson's disease. Most importantly, so far these approaches have been safe and have not caused any harm. In time, there will be more and more attempts to treat Parkinson's disease with gene therapy.

WHAT QUESTIONS DO I NEED TO ASK ABOUT NEUROSURGERY FOR PARKINSON'S SYMPTOMS?

Neurosurgical approaches for the treatment of Parkinson's disease are complex. There are many questions that people who have Parkinson's and their family members need to understand and explore when considering neurosurgery:

—Is my diagnosis of Parkinson's disease correct?

—Have I fully explored the medical (nonsurgical) alternatives?

—Is the surgical procedure effective for the symptoms responsible for my disability?

—How long can I expect the benefits of the surgery to last?

—Can I expect enough improvement to help my motor functioning?

—What types of patients are most likely to benefit from this procedure? Am I one of those types?

—Has the surgical procedure been perfected?

—What is the level of experience of my neurosurgeon and neurologist with this procedure?

—Aside from the neurologic effects, what effects is surgery likely to have on me? How uncomfortable will the procedure be, and how long will the discomfort last?

—What are the common adverse effects of this surgical procedure?

—What uncommon but serious complications have occurred or might be expected?

—Do I have problems that might make specific complications more likely or more serious?

—Will my medication regimen change after surgery?

—How much does the procedure cost, and is the cost covered by health insurance?

—Might this surgical procedure preclude other options in the future?

—Are my expectations realistic?

The only way to address all these very important questions is to consult a neurologist who has considerable experience with these procedures.

Go through the list with the neurologist. Speak to a neurosurgeon or another neurologist to get a second opinion (many health insurance plans require a second opinion before they will approve coverage of a surgical procedure). Be satisfied—or as satisfied as you can be—that you have good answers to your questions before you make a decision.

Part V

OTHER ISSUES

CHAPTER 17

Illness, Hospitalization, and Parkinson's Disease

- *How can a person who has Parkinson's disease ensure the best possible care when hospitalized?*
- *What medical complications are of particular concern to a person who has Parkinson's?*

People do not die directly from Parkinson's disease; however, advanced Parkinson's does increase the risk of problems, including serious conditions that may be life threatening, such as falls or infection. The most common reasons people who have Parkinson's disease must be hospitalized include elective surgery, falls with fractures, infections, a change in alertness (such as sleepiness, confusion, hallucinations), and aspiration pneumonia. We confine our discussion to what happens when he or she must enter the hospital for elective or emergency surgery or medical therapy.

Hospitals are large bureaucratic institutions, which, generally speaking, are not well suited to care for the needs of people who have Parkinson's disease. The hospital may be a first-rate institution in which coronary artery bypass surgery is performed, gallbladders are removed, and kidney ailments are treated. But it may be ineffective or lack experience in caring for the specific needs of people who have Parkinson's disease who are hospitalized. As long as the patient and family understand this, they can take necessary precautions to avoid common pitfalls of hospitalization for people who have Parkinson's disease.

MEDICATIONS IN THE HOSPITAL

One of the most common problems encountered when an individual who has Parkinson's is hospitalized involves his or her medication schedule. Members of the hospital staff are accustomed to administering medications on a 9 a.m., 1 p.m., 5 p.m., and 9 p.m. (or 9 a.m., 1 p.m., 5 p.m., and bedtime) schedule. As people who have Parkinson's disease know, their medication schedule is not that regimented or routine. They may well be taking medications every two to three hours, but individuals tend to work out their own schedule to get the most benefit from their antiparkinson medications. For example, they may find their medications work better if taken thirty minutes before meals, or twenty-five minutes before meals, or twelve minutes before meals.

If you are taking medication for Parkinson's symptoms and you are hospitalized for any reason, it's very unlikely that the hospital staff will be able to deliver your antiparkinson medications on the schedule you have found most effective. We know from experience that, given the pressures on staff, a complicated schedule of oral medications is simply not going to be followed with great accuracy. You may at first find it both disturbing and alarming that the staff is unable to do this, but rather than becoming increasingly upset with hospital staff for not delivering medications on schedule, you can take a proactive position. Discuss your complicated medication schedule with hospital staff at the time of admission. Inform them that it might be best if you and your family administer the antiparkinson medications yourselves rather than relying on hospital staff. This arrangement is usually possible. In this way, you can keep control of your own antiparkinson medications and better manage your symptoms while your other medical or surgical problems are attended to. Most important, be sure to tell your hospital physicians, house staff, and nursing staff precisely what medications you are taking and how much you are taking.

Another medication-related problem that often arises when a person who has Parkinson's is admitted to a general medical or surgical hospital ward is that she or he mistakenly receives drugs that conflict with antiparkinson medications, including a wide variety of drugs used to control behavior (see Chapter 13). It is important for the patient and family to monitor what medicines are being administered in the hospital, and for what reasons. This of course applies to *all* hospitalized patients, but people who have Parkinson's need to be particularly on the alert for medications that will make their Parkinson's symptoms worse.

The unfamiliarity of the hospital's medical or surgical floor staff with some of the unusual features of Parkinson's disease can create other problems. We have seen people who have Parkinson's who are not treated properly by hospital staff because the staff is unfamiliar with the problems of motor fluctuations. Many patients complain bitterly that staff members (of whatever medical or surgical service they are admitted to) refuse to help them in some of the activities of daily living such as dressing, showering, or eating.

Why is this happening? Because at another point during the day, staff members have seen the patient during an "on" period, when he or she is fully or nearly fully functional. This misunderstanding represents a serious gap in the education of the hospital staff, of course, but it is a gap that patients and their families need to know about. Then the patient and family can plan ahead to explain to the staff that at certain periods during the day, the patient may require more assistance or less assistance in carrying out some of the activities of daily living.

If you are hospitalized and you have motor fluctuations, there's nothing wrong in asking for help during a time when you are "off" and are unable to carry out certain functions. Again, letting staff know about the motor fluctuations in advance will help avoid misunderstanding and hurt feelings.

People who have Parkinson's and motor fluctuations also need to discuss the timing of their medications before and after elective surgery. Generally we recommend that whenever possible the surgery be scheduled for first thing in the morning. Patients should normally be allowed to take their first morning dose of medications with sips of water even if they are not to be taking anything by mouth on the day of the procedure. As long as the bowel has not been compromised and is functioning normally after the procedure most patients should be started back on their usual medication schedule immediately after surgery. In the case of bowel surgery, many patients cannot be restarted on medications immediately. Here it is very important for the doctors to plan in advance how to manage Parkinson medication control in the postoperative period, especially in patients who have moderate to severe Parkinson's disease and experience motor fluctuations. Patients and families should discuss this issue with their physicians in advance of elective surgery.

MEDICAL COMPLICATIONS

People who have Parkinson's disease are particularly susceptible to several specific medical complications when they are hospital inpatients. These medical complications sometimes cannot be avoided, but making sure that the internist, family practitioner, or surgeon is aware of this susceptibility may allow preventive measures to be taken. These problems include postoperative delirium, deep vein thrombosis (blood clots in the legs), and pneumonia.

Postoperative Delirium

Anyone who undergoes a medical or surgical procedure that requires the administration of a general anesthetic or considerable sedation is at risk for developing postoperative delirium or a confusional state. Postoperative confusion or delirium usually is self-limited, meaning it will disappear on its own within a short period of time, usually in one to three days. Patients with Parkinson's disease are somewhat more susceptible to the development of this problem, and everyone involved in the care of a person who has Parkinson's should be aware of this. This is particularly the case for patients who are elderly and those with preexisting cognitive problems. Any patient who is elderly or who has preexisting cognitive problems, whether they have Parkinson's disease or not, is potentially very sensitive to the use of narcotics for postoperative pain, and the use of these drugs in such patients should be avoided unless they are absolutely necessary. If at all possible, a procedure should be performed without the use of a general anesthetic (perhaps using, instead, a more local type of anesthesia). There are times, of course, when a local anesthetic is not appropriate and might be unsafe, and general anesthesia must be administered. If postprocedural confusion does develop, certain drugs should be avoided if possible, including some of those discussed in Chapter 13, which tend to make Parkinson's symptoms worse. Control of postoperative confusion should be managed very conservatively, generally by waiting for the problem to resolve itself, and medication to treat the confusion should be avoided if possible. If medications are essential, atypical neuroleptics such as quetiapine (Seroquel), or clozapine (Clozaril) should be used, and typical major tranquilizers such as haloperidol (commonly used for postoperative confusion in other patients) should definitely be avoided.

Postoperative-Procedure Nausea

It is not unusual for a person to feel nauseated after a surgical procedure, endoscopy, conscious sedation, or general anesthesia. Medications commonly used to control nausea and vomiting in these situations include prochlorperazine (Compazine) and metoclopramide (Reglan), both of which have dopamine antagonist activity. Because any medication that blocks or interferes with brain dopamine activity will worsen Parkinson's disease, these medications should be avoided in people who have Parkinson's disease. Another antinausea/vomiting medication that will not worsen parkinsonism and that is quite effective is odansetron (Zofran). It is best to speak to your surgeon, proceduralist, or internist in advance about this potential problem.

Deep Vein Thrombosis

Deep vein thrombosis (blood clots in the veins) tends to develop in the muscles of the legs when people are immobile for long periods. People who have Parkinson's have an added problem, of course: immobility is a characteristic of their illness, and with the additional immobility imposed by the recovery time after a surgical procedure, the risk of deep vein thrombosis or clots increases. If you are to undergo surgery, discuss this problem with the physician admitting you to the hospital. Methods are available to help prevent blood clots in the lower extremities, including physical therapy and certain medications. An aggressive program to prevent deep vein thrombosis is of value to hospitalized patients with Parkinson's disease. If deep vein thrombosis does occur, treatment consists of blood-thinning medications and very careful monitoring. The threat is that the clot will break loose and travel to the lungs, and this must be avoided.

Pneumonia

All patients are at risk for developing pneumonia after a surgical procedure. However, people who have Parkinson's may be at greater risk because they sometimes have more difficulty generating the deep coughing necessary to prevent accumulation of fluid in the lungs. A person who has Parkinson's must receive detailed instructions over and above the usual instructions given by the respiratory therapist for postoperative management of the lungs. More time should be spent explaining what will need to be done postoperatively and the importance of deep coughing and the other exercises prescribed by respiratory therapists.

Another type of pneumonia that some people who have Parkinson's may be prone to is aspiration pneumonia, as discussed in Chapter 5. This type of pneumonia results from a swallowing dysfunction in which food, which is supposed to go down the esophagus into the stomach, enters the lungs. There are many precautions the hospital staff can take to prevent aspiration pneumonia in a patient who is at risk. Once again, be sure to ask your internist and surgeon whether special measures are needed to prevent aspiration in your particular case.

RECOVERY

Generally speaking, people who have Parkinson's disease will require lengthier hospitalizations for the same illness or injury than people the same age who do not have Parkinson's disease. If more attention was paid to proper timing of Parkinson's medication in the hospital, more judicious use was made of antinausea agents, and careful attention was paid to preventing aspiration, the length of stay in the hospital could be shortened.

Finally, recovery time is generally longer for people who have Parkinson's disease. Physicians often give patients an estimate of how long it will take them to recover from a particular procedure or surgical operation. For example, the surgeon may tell someone that after an elective procedure, they will need six weeks to get "back to normal." The rule of thumb is that a person who has Parkinson's disease takes two to three times longer than a person without Parkinson's to recover from any surgical procedure. The body simply takes longer to readjust to its baseline activities in a person who has Parkinson's disease. Thus, whatever medical or surgical procedure you are to undergo, if you have Parkinson's disease you will have a more prolonged period of recuperation. This is nothing to be concerned about. It simply has to be planned for.

CHAPTER 18

Parkinson's Disease Research

- *What are the active areas of research in Parkinson's disease?*
- *Why does scientific progress take so long?*
- *How can people who have Parkinson's and their families help?*

Some promising leads are being followed by scientists and physicians developing new treatments for people who have Parkinson's disease. But the pace of clinical research can seem excruciatingly slow for a person who has a progressive disorder such as Parkinson's. In this chapter we describe some of this research and how it is conducted, so that people who have Parkinson's and their families have a better understanding of why new discoveries and new treatments require such a long time to become widely available. We also return to a discussion begun in Chapter 1 about the possibility of patients' participation in clinical trials, and look at some other ways people who have Parkinson's disease and their families can help.

BASIC AND CLINICAL RESEARCH

Scientific research is labor intensive, time consuming, and costly. Although not evident to the person who has Parkinson's, the pace of progress in the management of this disease has been relatively rapid— especially considering the obstacles that had to be overcome along the way. The fact is that there are no shortcuts to sound scientific discovery. Progress can be made only through trial and error, multiple tests, and the painstaking demonstration that a new drug, surgical procedure, or complementary therapy for Parkinson's disease is safe and effective. In this section we review the steps that must be followed to develop discovery into therapy.

The processes of discovery and development that are the hallmarks of both *basic research*, conducted by scientists, and *clinical research*, conducted by clinical researchers (physicians), are collaborative efforts in which scientists and physicians continually interact. Both basic and clinical research involve a delicate balancing act, as well: the urgency to discover remedies, even cures, for disabling illness balanced by the requirement to avoid posing risk to the patient by proceeding with caution and paying attention to every detail; and the vast financial investment required for research balanced by the potential for windfall profits from an important discovery. Basic research is funded both by the government and by pharmaceutical companies; clinical research is more often funded by pharmaceutical companies.

Basic Research

When doing basic scientific research in the biological sciences, investigators explore biological processes that may or may not have a relationship to disease. Fundamental basic research involves working at the cellular level (for example using various types of cells in culture), known as *in vitro* research, and working in living animals, known as *in vivo* research. Important discoveries usually entail studies in both these categories of research. Although a new understanding of a fundamental biological process may, in fact, have profound implications for understanding a disease process, researchers generally cannot predict whether research in a basic biological area will have practical or clinical application. For this reason, it is not always clear where time, money, and effort should be spent.

For example, no one could have predicted that the initial investigation of the neurochemistry of the cow brain would lead to fundamental discoveries about Parkinson's disease. Yet a new understanding of the potential role of dopamine in the brain resulted from the discovery that dopamine occurs in high concentrations in the basal ganglia of the cow brain. And this finding subsequently led to the discovery that dopamine levels are reduced in the basal ganglia of people who have Parkinson's disease and, eventually, to replacement therapy with levodopa.

While many scientific discoveries rely on serendipity such as this, important breakthroughs have also come from careful planning and following a "hunch" based on many tantalizing scientific clues. Because government funding for basic research has become increasingly competitive, researchers are increasingly being asked to demonstrate in advance a strong likelihood that their research project will lead to the development of practical applications. Funding is generally awarded to projects that appear to have a greater chance of practical application (although, as noted above, it's often difficult to tell in advance whether this will prove to be the case). This type of focused basic research often grows out of conversations between basic scientists and clinical physicians. The physician highlights the practical needs of patients, and the scientist is motivated by this information to move into areas of serious need.

There is great interest in the possibility of using *stem cells* for treating Parkinson's disease. Stem cells are a type of cell that has the potential, under the right biological conditions, to develop into any type of adult body cell. A stem cell may become a neuron (say, in the brain) or a kidney cell or a heart muscle cell, and so on. The hope for the usefulness of stem cells in Parkinson's is that a supply of brain cells that produce dopamine (the chemical whose absence is responsible for many features of the disease) would be readily available to transplant into the brain of people who have Parkinson's. If this were successful, this type of therapy might actually be neurorestorative or neuroregenerative. In other words, this therapy might repair some of the damage already caused in the brain by Parkinson's disease.

Stem cells can be harvested from human embryos or from certain adult tissues. There is considerable scientific confusion at this early stage of the investigation as to which source of stem cells is preferable. Unfortunately, in the United States there has been a great deal of political controversy over access to stem cells. Because of the enormous public interest in stem cells (i.e., in the possibility of important therapeutic advances in many fields of medicine besides Parkinson's), some states (California and Maryland, among others) have begun state-funded initiatives to circumvent the federal government's restrictions on stem cell research. In recent years, the political climate in the United States has made investigation using stem cells easier.

All the political machinations aside, investigation into the therapeutic use of stem cells is in its infancy, and whether or not there is any real therapeutic potential for people who have Parkinson's disease is completely unknown at this time. It is important for people who have Parkinson's not to put all their hopes in stem cells, since so many scientific hurdles have yet to be crossed before we even get to the stage of beginning clinical trials of stem cells in Parkinson's disease.

Animal Testing

When basic research leads to a discovery with potential importance for clinical work, investigators use animal testing to determine whether a new treatment is safe and effective for testing in humans. Discovery of a neurochemical that appears to have some benefit in an animal model of a disease process triggers numerous stages of further animal testing before the chemical is tested as a drug in patients with a specific disease.

When people read in a newspaper article or hear on the television news that a new drug has been found to improve symptoms in an animal model of Parkinson's disease, they often don't realize that many more stages of animal testing are required before the drug is tested on humans. In animal testing, the drug is tested for potential *effectiveness* and for *toxicity*. Toxicologic tests are especially important to evaluate whether a new drug may damage such organs as the liver, kidney, or heart or has the potential to cause cancer.

Although the preliminary stages of testing appear promising, the new drug announced in the news will not be available for clinical trials in people who have Parkinson's disease for several years. And even if the drug is found to be safe and effective in animals and then proves safe and effective in clinical research in Parkinson's patients, many years of human testing will be required to gather additional information before the U.S. Food and Drug Administration (FDA), the regulatory agency for new drugs in the United States, approves the drug for use in humans.

Clinical Trials

If the drug passes the toxicologic tests, it moves on to being tested in normal, healthy, young human volunteers. (Tests involving humans are called *clinical trials*.) The first tests of a drug in humans are done in healthy individuals, and they are done to evaluate *safety* only (so-called Phase I studies). Investigators conducting the trials for the pharmaceutical company sponsoring the research look for symptoms such as low blood pressure, increased heart rate, excessive nausea, or dizziness, which would make the drug unsafe for use in the patient population.

If the drug passes the testing phase in healthy volunteers, it moves into the initial stages of evaluation in a relatively small number of people who have Parkinson's disease. These early trials of a drug in people who have disease are conducted under very carefully controlled conditions (Phase II studies). Participants may be admitted to the hospital for drug testing and monitoring, or they may be required to make very frequent visits to the neurologist. A drug that passes these stages of close monitoring for *safety* and *effectiveness* may proceed to larger, multi-institutional clinical research trials (Phase III trials). Once the drug is finally marketed, the studies done after marketing are classified as Phase IV studies. Generally Phase II and III studies involve random allocation of patients to either the active drug (sometimes in different doses) or a placebo. Sometimes in Phase III studies the drug of interest is compared to another active drug known to be effective in Parkinson's disease (a so-called active comparator).

The pharmaceutical company developing a drug for Parkinson's disease needs to conduct trials to prove safety and effectiveness in specific situations. For example, one study might be designed to look at how well the drug is tolerated by, and how effective it is, in people recently diagnosed with Parkinson's. A separate study might be designed to look at individuals with more advanced symptoms. Any hints of problems related to the new drug precipitate extensive further testing and analysis—or discontinuation of trials altogether.

All clinical research on human beings must be supervised and approved by an *institutional review board*. Institutional review boards carefully examine any study plan, or protocol, to assure that guidelines for safety and ethical conduct of research are being observed. They also make sure that the investigators obtain a fully informed consent from each person enrolled in the study. The institutional review board requires investigators to submit periodic updates about the progress of the people in the study. If there is any reason to believe that the study participants are at unnecessary or inappropriate risk, the board has the authority to intervene and withdraw approval.

Once the clinical trials have been completed, the pharmaceutical company submits the extensive data collected from the trials to a government regulatory agency, such as the FDA in the United States or its counterparts in other countries. The regulatory agency then reviews all the data to determine whether they have been collected properly, whether the data and statistical analyses are valid, and whether the drug has any serious side effects or unacceptable risks. After much deliberation and scrutiny, the FDA issues a ruling on whether the drug is approved for marketing—whether it can now be prescribed for use by people with disease.

As noted above, the entire procedure—from the discovery of a biological process that may be important to a disease process, through all the animal and human studies, to FDA approval—requires many years of work, and the costs involved are enormous. Some people argue that the process currently takes too long, and undoubtedly some efforts could be made toward streamlining some of the steps. There is a danger, however, in short-circuiting this process: drugs with questionable effectiveness or safety could be put on the market. The objective is to maintain a critical balance between scientific progress and patient safety.

PROMISING AVENUES OF RESEARCH IN PARKINSON'S DISEASE

Research into Parkinson's disease has many promising avenues, many promising developments that may bear fruit in the coming years. One area of enormous interest is the use of new types of imaging to "see" the brain in Parkinson's disease. Significant progress is being made in our ability to look at the brain with new techniques, including

PET (positron emission tomography), SPECT (single photon emission computed tomography), new approaches to MRI (magnetic resonance imaging), and transcranial sonography. The research into each of these techniques may well lead to a test for the diagnosis of Parkinson's disease, more accurate information about the progress of the illness in a specific individual, and a greater ability to distinguish among all the "cousins" of Parkinson's disease. The SPECT Scan (DATScan), previously available in Europe, is now available in the United States and is being used to distinguish between essential tremor (see Chapter 10) and parkinsonism. Unfortunately, there is still no imaging technique that can distinguish between the "cousins" of Parkinson's disease. Transcranial sonography is widely used in Europe, particularly in Germany; it has not been adopted in the United Kingdom, Canada, or the United States, although some centers are beginning to get experience with this technique.

In addition to research in diagnostic technology, current studies are devoted both to discovering the cause of Parkinson's, which could lead to preventive measures, and to developing new treatments for the symptoms of the disease, including complementary therapies.

Finding the Cause of Parkinson's Disease

As noted in Chapter 2, it appears highly unlikely that Parkinson's disease is caused exclusively by a person's genetic makeup or exclusively by an environmental toxin. But research in both epidemiology (the study of the incidence, distribution, and control of a disease in a population) and genetics is ongoing and vigorous, as is research into what causes nerve cells (neurons) to become damaged and die. All these avenues of research into disease causation must be followed, not only to avoid overlooking any possible means of preventing Parkinson's but also to explore the widest possible range of approaches to therapy for people who have the disease.

Epidemiology. Researchers in the field of epidemiology are focusing their efforts on searching for "common threads" among the different individuals who develop Parkinson's disease. They are looking at the lifestyles of patients—what they eat, where they live, the type of water they drink, and the types of pesticides or industrial toxins they may have been exposed to—as well as their family history.

As noted in Chapter 2, studies of twins may also be useful in helping epidemiologists determine who gets Parkinson's disease, and why. Let's suppose a disease is determined purely by a single gene. For identical twins, we would expect that if one of the pair developed the disease, the other twin would develop it too. For fraternal twins (who do not share identical genes), if one twin developed the disease, the other twin would be only as likely to develop it as any other sibling of the twins. If one identical twin develops Parkinson's symptoms and the other does not, it suggests that nongenetic factors may be more important than genetic factors in causing the disease—perhaps the twin with Parkinson's was exposed to a toxin in the environment that the unaffected twin did not encounter. Unfortunately, we are learning that things are never as simple or as straightforward as originally conceived. The field of epigenetics is now teaching us that identical twins are not as genetically identical as was once believed, so interpretation of twin studies may be more difficult than previously thought.

Genetics. A very active area of research is the evaluation of genetics in Parkinson's disease. Asked whether they have any family members with Parkinson's, the large majority of people with the disease say no. However, several studies have found a greater risk of the illness in family members of people who have Parkinson's disease. In 1996, quite a stir was generated in the scientific community by the discovery of a gene responsible for parkinsonism in a large Italian family (see Chapter 2) and three smaller Greek families (the gene mutation probably originated in Greece and was then transported to Italy through naval traffic centuries ago). The syndromes in these family members have enough in common with Parkinson's disease to raise the question of whether the same gene or similar genes are affected in people who have Parkinson's.

The members of these Italian and Greek families are somewhat different from the average person who has Parkinson's disease. First of all, these families have a very high prevalence of illness in each generation, with half or more of the family members in a single generation affected by parkinsonism. In addition, the onset of the disorder occurs at a much younger age in some family members than is usual for Parkinson's disease. Researchers have discovered that the gene found in the Italian family produces a protein, α-synuclein, known to occur in Lewy bodies, structures found at autopsy in the brains of people who have Parkinson's disease. While numerous unsuccessful attempts have been made to find a gene responsible for Parkinson's in the general population, the finding of a single gene in a single family has led to important fundamental knowledge about Parkinson's disease (see Chapter 2).

Since this original discovery, researchers have found more genes to be of potential importance in several different families with more typical Parkinson's disease and other genes in people who have young-onset parkinsonism. These "new" genes include Parkin, DJ-1, PINK1, and LRRK2. The discovery of these genes that are linked to parkinsonism has led to rethinking the possible genetic basis of Parkinson's disease. Rather startlingly for experienced Parkinson's doctors, these gene mutations result in a clinical picture (phenotype) that cannot be distinguished from sporadic adult onset Parkinson's disease. This raises the question of how many more specific gene mutations that resulted in Parkinson's disease will be discovered.

The genetics revolution in Parkinson's disease is paralleled by rapid advances in technology of gene discovery. It has become feasible to survey the entire human genome looking for clues to Parkinson's disease. This is a rapidly burgeoning field that is yielding new results virtually every week. It has also led to a new problem in Parkinson's disease research, which is how to be sure whether the "new" genes being discovered actually play a role in the development of Parkinson's disease. This dilemma has led to a novel approach: results of genome-wide association studies (looking at a patient's entire genome) are paired with inserting the discovered genes in a fly (Drosophila) model to test whether or not they have functional significance. This is a simple, elegant model, and we think it will yield remarkable results in the years ahead.

Research into the Mechanisms of Cell Damage. Finding out what causes progressive nerve cell damage and death and what that process involves is important because in Parkinson's disease, nerve cells are damaged and die regardless of what starts that process (e.g., a combination of genetics and an environmental toxin). There may be many different triggers but a limited number of final pathways or processes that eventually cause nerve cells to degenerate. Because of this, the study of *neuroprotection* is an important area of research for Parkinson's disease and many other neurologic disorders. Neuroprotection refers to the concept that a drug might be capable of stopping or slowing the progression of the disease process. If such a drug existed, we would not need to know the cause of Parkinson's disease in order to alter its progress.

The hope is that a neuroprotective agent would slow down the clock, so symptoms currently expected to appear after five to ten years of illness would not appear until much later, say after fifteen or twenty years. At the present time, no such drug exists. Researchers continue to study various cellular systems within the brain to determine possible mechanisms for neuroprotection.

An important part of developing effective neuroprotective therapy is to establish more accurate and reliable animal models of this progressive neurodegenerative disease. Another priority in the search for neuroprotection is to find reliable "biomarkers" that can provide a more accurate and earlier diagnosis and can track the progression of the disease more reliably than simple clinical exams and the currently available imaging techniques.

As discussed in Chapter 16, using *neurotrophic factors*—the natural body chemicals that promote the growth and survival of brain cells— as neuroprotective agents is another important avenue of study. Neurotrophic factors may well improve survival of, or even promote recovery of, injured areas of the brain. The large effort under way to improve our understanding of the basic aging process is also likely to yield important breakthroughs in the area of neuroprotection.

Finding New Approaches to Symptomatic Therapy

Medications. While a symptomatic drug does not alter the progression of the disease, it often significantly alters the symptoms of the disease and markedly improves a person's quality of life. As noted throughout this book, many symptomatic medications are available for

Parkinson's disease, but the currently available therapy still has many weaknesses. Medications with improved effectiveness, fewer and less severe side effects, and greater convenience would be welcome.

Some Parkinson's symptoms are only partly relieved by current therapy, and a number of symptoms are still poorly responsive to any currently available intervention. Symptoms that may only partly respond include tremor, freezing while walking, loss of balance, and motor fluctuations. Symptoms such as constipation, depression, urinary incontinence, speech difficulty, and sexual dysfunction also may not respond adequately to available medications in individual patients. Cognitive dysfunction continues to be one of the most difficult problems to treat, and there is an urgent need for improved therapies in this area.

People who have Parkinson's disease would also benefit from the discovery of symptomatic medications with less tendency to provoke side effects such as dyskinesia, hallucinations, nausea, dizziness, and sleepiness. And because pill schedules can be demanding and intrusive, medications that offer greater convenience would include longer-acting medications that reduce dosing frequency or skin patches that provide more continuous medication delivery with less bother. Skin patches for Parkinson's disease have been effective in clinical trials. Rotigotine (formerly marketed as Neupro) is an example of a dopamine agonist delivered by skin patch. Although this patch was effective in both early and advanced Parkinson's disease and was preferred by many patients, the internal drug properties of the patch resulted in the drug crystallizing in the patch. The company withdrew the patch and developed a new noncrystallizing patch that is again marketed in the United States and Europe.

Surgery. As discussed in Chapter 16, neurosurgical procedures are a significant avenue of clinical research today. We do not know what role these procedures will ultimately play in the management of Parkinson's disease. Will they prove so safe and effective that they take the place of medications? Or will they continue to be used for the smaller subgroup of people who have advanced symptoms that cannot be relieved by medication? We won't know the full answers to these questions for years to come. This question is still not answered. Most researchers are hopeful that new discoveries will ultimately put deep brain stimulation (DBS) "out of business," the idea being that if something better (a medication) is discovered, the need for invasive surgery will be eliminated. Having made that point, however, we still can say that DBS surgery for Parkinson's disease has been an enormous advance in the treatment of Parkinson's disease (see Chapter 16).

Exercise and Rehabilitation Therapy. As discussed in Chapter 14, investigating the effects of physical and cognitive training on the symptoms of Parkinson's disease is an increasingly important area of research. These approaches are unique in an important way: they are effective interventions that people who have Parkinson's disease can do to help themselves. There is something especially empowering and energizing when the person who has a chronic condition can take matters in their own hands and do something about it. Initiating and maintaining a routine of physical training is not a substitute for the important pharmacologic and surgical therapies that address symptoms, but it is a necessary and effective supplement to achieve the very best outcomes over time. There is still much to learn about exercise and rehabilitation in Parkinson's disease. Some of the most pressing questions include: What are the effects of combinations of different types of exercise? What types of exercise are most effective at the different stages of Parkinson's disease? Is it possible to delay disability and even the underlying changes in the brain with physical and cognitive training?

Complementary Therapies. We conclude our discussion of research directions for the relief of Parkinson's disease symptoms with an area that is virtually neglected by current research efforts: complementary or alternative therapies (see Chapter 15). These therapies are gaining increasing public acceptance, despite the few sources of funding for research into the safety or effectiveness of these approaches.

As noted in Chapter 15, unlike medications, which are regulated by the FDA, alternative therapies can be marketed for a range of disorders without any proof of effectiveness. As the proportion of the health care dollar allocated to alternative therapies steadily grows, research efforts to prove or disprove claims of effectiveness are necessary. The government will most likely have to step in and enact regulations to provide adequate scrutiny of alternative therapies. In the United States, new regulations concerning dietary supplements and claims about their effectiveness already have been introduced. Whether or not the new regulations alter the marketing of dietary supplements remains to be seen. The Division of Intramural Research of the National Center for Complementary and Alternative Medicine, part of the National Institutes of Health (NIH), constitutes an effort to address this growing problem. In our view, in the future there should be no such thing as "alternative medicine"—there should only be "medicine," all of which has been studied and proven to work or not.

PATIENTS AND FAMILIES
HELPING THE RESEARCH EFFORT

People who have Parkinson's disease and their families and friends can help in the research process in three ways. First, individuals with Parkinson's can participate in clinical research trials. We often explain to our patients who have early, mild, or advanced disease that any medication that is helpful to them now or in the future is available only because other patients and families participated in research trials before them. People who have Parkinson's disease and their caregivers form a community, and the only way progress can be made is for people to consider taking part in the process that results in that progress. Of course, people have no guarantee that participating in a clinical research trial will benefit them directly. But even beyond those instances where a new drug, surgical technique, or device proves useful (in which case the participant will have had early access to the treatment), the evidence suggests that simply taking part in a research trial produces emotional and physical benefits—in no small measure because of the high level of medical monitoring of individuals enrolled in clinical trials.

Second, patients and families can help by being involved with the political and social forces that shape the policies and funding procedures of state and federal governments. The political will of patients' commitment can be very effective in directing revenues to a significant national health problem such as Parkinson's. People interested in pursuing this important work can become involved in a Parkinson's disease organization or foundation, and they can write letters or send email messages to their representatives at the state and federal levels, explaining the importance of health services and research in Parkinson's disease.

Finally, because of growing competition for the limited funding available from the government, private donations and contributions to help support basic and clinical research are extremely important. This is a delicate issue, and we understand that individuals have different financial resources and commitments, but people are often surprised to discover how helpful private donations are to the support of costly research activities. Contributions can be made to a specific Parkinson's disease organization (see Resources) or to any of the Parkinson's disease programs located at most major medical schools in the United States and Canada.

CHAPTER 19

Questions and Answers

In this chapter we answer some questions that many patients, families, and caregivers have asked us about Parkinson's disease. In the answers, we also direct you to the chapter or chapters in this book that have a complete discussion of the topic.

DEFINITIONS AND BASICS

Q: What is Parkinson's disease?

A: Parkinson's disease is a progressive neurodegenerative disorder that affects a specific group of nerve cells in the brain. This group of cells, called the substantia nigra, uses the neurotransmitter dopamine to communicate within the brain. In people who have Parkinson's disease, the cells of the substantia nigra progressively die, or degenerate, and this is accompanied by a loss of dopamine. It is this progressive loss of cells in the substantia nigra with loss of dopamine that leads to the dominant symptoms of Parkinson's disease (Chapter 1). These symptoms include resting tremor (rhythmical shaking), rigidity (stiffness of muscles), bradykinesia and akinesia (slowness of movement and lack of movement), and loss of postural reflexes (difficulty with balance) (Chapters 3, 4, and 5). Parkinson's disease is much more than just a dopamine deficiency disorder, and managing the symptoms that are not related to too little dopamine remains a challenge, especially in the later stages of the disease. We do not know the cause of Parkinson's disease. At this time there is no cure for Parkinson's, but a wide variety of medications are helpful in relieving the symptoms of the disease (Chapters 12 and 13).

Q: Why me?

A: This is an understandable question, and a question that most people ask many times when first diagnosed with Parkinson's disease: why have I been singled out for this disorder? The answer is that we don't know of any clear predisposing factors for Parkinson's disease. In other words, there is no answer to the question of why a specific individual develops this disorder (Chapter 2).

Q: Will other members of my family develop Parkinson's disease?

A: For the most part, Parkinson's disease is not a familial disorder. The large majority of people who have Parkinson's are not aware of other family members having the disease. Although the evidence for heredity as a factor in developing Parkinson's disease is not strong, there is considerable new evidence that in a small number of families, an abnormal gene can cause parkinsonism. Even in those families where a genetic abnormality is found, however, other factors most likely play an important role in determining whether this genetic factor is expressed as disease, and at what age. When one member of a family is affected with Parkinson's disease, close relatives may have a slightly greater risk of developing Parkinson's than does the population at large (Chapter 2).

Q: Is it infectious?

A: No. You cannot catch Parkinson's disease from being close to or taking care of someone with Parkinson's.

Q: What is "symptomatic therapy" for Parkinson's disease?

A: All of the medications discussed in this book that help alleviate the basic problems experienced by people who have Parkinson's disease—such as tremor, stiffness, slowness, balance, and walking problems—are called symptomatic treatments. These medications help with the symptoms and signs of Parkinson's but do not treat the underlying cause of the disease. The cause of Parkinson's disease is unknown, and we do not have any treatments that change or slow the disease process (Chapters 12 and 13).

Q: What is "neuroprotective therapy" for Parkinson's disease?

A: Neuroprotective therapy is a treatment for Parkinson's disease that would modify or slow the progression of the disease. This is a very important concept, and many clinical research trials are investigating a variety of drugs that have the potential to achieve this effect. Slowing disease progression would be very helpful to people who have Parkinson's and would be a wonderful advance in treatment. Unfortunately, there is currently no proven neuroprotective agent (Chapters 13 and 18).

Q: What is "disease-modifying" therapy for Parkinson's disease?

A: A disease-modifying therapy is any treatment modality—medications; physical, occupational, or speech therapy; exercise program; or surgery—that "modifies" the known course of the disease. The term "disease modifying" is being used as a new approach or new response to treatment that changes the course of the disease. In some ways it is similar to a symptomatic treatment but in contrast to a symptomatic treatment, if a successful disease-modifying therapy were stopped it is expected that the patient would *not* lose the benefit over a short period of time, as would be expected if the patient were to stop a purely symptomatic treatment. The term "disease modifying" was introduced to acknowledge that treatments that, it is hoped, are neuroprotective may not have a direct effect on nerve cell degeneration but may nevertheless influence the natural course of the disease in other ways. For example, there are a number of ways that the brain tries to compensate for the loss of dopamine (other cells become more active, or dopamine receptors increase their avidity for dopamine). These compensatory mechanisms probably fail over time (accounting in part for how and when patients' symptoms become evident). A disease-modifying therapy might somehow restore or bolster some of these failing functions, thus improving the course of the disease without having any impact at all on the dopamine neuronal degeneration.

Q: What is "neurorestorative/neuroregenerative therapy" for Parkinson's disease?

A: Neurorestorative/neuroregenerative therapy is any treatment that would "reverse" the damage, replace damaged tissue, or restore normal function in certain areas of the brain in a person who has Parkinson's disease. This type of therapy is probably closest to what people have in mind when they speak of a cure. Much basic and clinical research is taking place in this area, but at present there is no proven neurorestorative/neuroregenerative treatment.

PROGNOSIS

Q: What is the prognosis for someone with Parkinson's disease?
A: The prognosis varies among individuals. Because Parkinson's is a progressive disorder, however, a person who has this disease will probably notice some additional, small problem each year, despite treatment. Many people who have Parkinson's do extremely well for years, maintaining a high quality of life twelve to fifteen years into the illness, whereas other people have a great deal of motor difficulty within five to ten years of the onset of the disorder. At present we have no way to predict how quickly significant impairment will develop for any individual. There is some evidence that people whose Parkinson's disease is tremor predominant—in other words, tremor is more apparent than slowness or rigidity (called akinetic, or rigid predominant) may have slower progression of motor symptoms.

Q: What should I expect to happen to me in the first two to three years after I'm diagnosed with Parkinson's disease?
A: Following the emergence of the first symptoms of Parkinson's disease, the next two to three years after the initial diagnosis should be reasonably stable, with slight increases in severity of the symptoms, including perhaps an increase in tremor, some increase in slowness, or mild changes in walking habits. Medications will work very well to alleviate these problems, and you should have no significant disability, no cognitive dysfunction, and no significant disturbance of balance at this time (Chapter 3).

Q: How do the symptoms usually progress?
A: After a period of three to five years, stronger or higher doses of antiparkinson medication will probably be required to control the symptoms. Medications generally are highly effective for the emerging

symptoms, and people usually continue to do reasonably well. From four to seven years after the diagnosis or onset of the disease, people may begin to experience some of the complications related to long-term antiparkinson drug therapy, including periods of "wearing-off" of medication effects, mild dyskinesia (involuntary movements), or infrequent nonthreatening visual hallucinations. The ability to perform the activities of daily living is likely to be affected (Chapter 4).

Major parkinsonian disability is rarely seen until after seven years, and significant disability usually does not occur until later than that (Chapter 5). Often the level of disability or difficulty in performing activities varies from hour to hour, depending upon when medication was last taken. Functional status, or functioning, may be excellent (possibly even normal or near normal) when the medication is working (during the "on" period), with periodic disability as the medication wears off (the "off" period) (Chapter 12).

Q: Will I be an invalid?

A: Again, the disease follows a unique course in every individual. At this time, we have no way to predict the course of disease severity in a specific person who has Parkinson's disease. Some people who have Parkinson's do eventually become dependent on others for the activities of daily living, such as dressing, going to the bathroom, and feeding, but many do not (Chapter 5).

Q: What is the relationship between Parkinson's disease and Alzheimer's disease?

A: Parkinson's disease and Alzheimer's disease are two separate disease processes. The symptoms of early Parkinson's are largely due to involvement a specific area deep within the brain called the substantia nigra, whereas Alzheimer's involves the cerebral cortex, a larger area of the brain located near the surface, as well as some deeper structures. The initial symptoms of the two disorders are markedly different as well (Chapter 10). However, with time, some people who have Alzheimer's do get "motor" symptoms that can sometimes be confused with parkinsonism, and some people who have Parkinson's disease can develop cognitive dysfunction that could be confused with Alzheimer's.

Q: What is the relationship between Parkinson's and normal pressure hydrocephalus (NPH)?

A: Normal pressure hydrocephalus is a relatively rare condition in which the fluid-filled spaces in the brain (the ventricles) become enlarged. When this happens in an older individual, a triad of symptoms may emerge consisting of a gait abnormality (often called a *magnetic gait,* because it appears that the person's feet are glued to the floor); urinary problems progressing to incontinence; and mild to moderate cognitive or thinking changes. Sometimes, people who have NPH also develop mild parkinsonism (rigidity, slowness, shuffling of gait). There are several signs that your doctor can use to distinguish NPH from Parkinson's. Brain imaging (obtained using CT scan or MRI scan) demonstrates marked enlargement of the ventricles in a person who has normal pressure hydrocephalus, while brain imaging is usually normal in Parkinson's or could show loss of brain substance (atrophy) related to age. The treatment for NPH is entirely different from that for Parkinson's (Chapters 8, 9, and 10).

Q: Does stress make the symptoms of Parkinson's disease worse?

A: Stress can temporarily aggravate symptoms of Parkinson's disease, but it does not affect the underlying progression of the disease. In other words, if someone is very anxious, under pressure, angry, or excited, the Parkinson's tremor will worsen. Slowness and gait difficulty may also get worse. When the stress or excitement passes, however, tremor, slowness, and gait problems return to their baseline level. For some people, a period of unusual stress may reveal the tremor somewhat earlier than it would have appeared otherwise, but the Parkinson's disease symptoms would have appeared eventually, even if this stressful event had not intervened. Stress does not cause or permanently worsen Parkinson's disease.

FOOD, DRINK, AND EXERCISE

Q: What activities and foods should I avoid?

A: No activities or foods are specifically prohibited for people who have Parkinson's disease. We strongly encourage physical activity and exercise to your level of tolerance, both in early and more advanced disease (Chapter 14). There are no special dietary restrictions for a person who has Parkinson's. Much attention has been focused on the protein redistribution diet, and this diet may be helpful for people who experience motor fluctuations while taking carbidopa/levodopa (Sinemet or Sinemet CR) (Chapters 12 and 13).

Q: Can I still drink alcohol with Parkinson's disease?

A: Under any circumstances, alcohol should be consumed in moderation and using good sense. There is no medical reason why a person who has Parkinson's disease cannot have a beer, a cocktail, or a glass of wine. In fact, the relaxing qualities of alcohol can be beneficial for symptoms, particularly tremor. All antiparkinson medications are compatible with a moderate amount of alcohol. Alcohol does have a multiplying effect on the sedative properties of drugs taken to treat anxiety or sleep problems (the benzodiazepines, including Valium, Tranxene, Xanax, Ativan, Restoril, and Klonopin), so if you are taking any of these drugs, use caution in drinking alcohol and be aware of excessive drowsiness.

WORK AND LEISURE ACTIVITIES

Q: How long should I continue to work?

A: Job and career can be an important source of satisfaction, and most people do not make the decision to discontinue employment lightly. Following the diagnosis of Parkinson's disease, the decision about whether to continue working depends upon several factors: personality, ability to perform the job, financial considerations, the wish to enjoy a period of retirement with a good quality of life, employment benefits (such as mental stimulation and social contacts), and the amount of stress resulting from the job and the work schedule. Ultimately, the decision to continue work or not depends on whether you feel that work enhances or detracts from your quality of life (Chapter 1).

Q: Will I still be able to drive my car?

A: Having Parkinson's disease does not mean that you can't drive a car, but it is important to realize that Parkinson's may seriously compromise your ability to drive safely. The motor disability of Parkinson's disease, including slow motor responses (the inability to respond quickly to changing situations) and excessive tremor, dyskinesia, or freezing, may be incompatible with controlling a motor vehicle. The cognitive dysfunction that sometimes appears in more advanced Parkinson's disease can make driving a car dangerous. Excessive daytime sleepiness caused by medications can also affect a person's ability to drive safely. Common sense dictates that you should err on the side of caution in this serious matter of driving.

When there is doubt or disagreement, a professional driving evaluator can assess a person's driving skills using a specially equipped vehicle to ensure safety in the testing situation. Loss of the independence that driving provides is an emotionally charged issue, and accepting this change is sometimes easier if the recommendation comes after an in-depth assessment of a person's driving abilities has shown that he or she is simply not able to drive as safely as necessary.

Q: Will I be able to travel?

A: For many people travel is an enriching experience, and there is no reason why a person who has Parkinson's disease cannot travel. People who have early or moderate Parkinson's disease generally experience no difficulty in traveling. People who have more advanced Parkinson's and increased disability need to consider their special needs when making travel plans. Consider your limitations when planning your vacation, and don't schedule more activities, or more strenuous activities, than you can enjoy. Make any medication adjustments well before starting out—don't start new medications or attempt to alter dosages while on vacation. It is especially important to keep several days' supply of drugs with you in a handbag or carryall, rather than placing all of your medication in luggage that may become lost in transit.

Q: When traveling across time zones, should I adjust my medication schedule?

A: People who have few or no motor fluctuations should simply take their medication using the time of their current time zone. For example, flights from the United States or Canada to Europe tend to leave in the afternoon or evening. If you are taking such a flight, follow your usual medication schedule at home that day and then resume your medication schedule using the new time upon arrival at your destination. People who have motor fluctuations, whose level of functioning is closely linked to the precision of their medication timing, may need to take more or less medication (depending on the direction of travel) on the day of travel to a distant time zone. Discuss this with your doctor before you travel.

Q: Are antiparkinson medications available in other countries?

A: Antiparkinson medications, especially the various forms of carbidopa/levodopa, are available throughout the world. Of course, in other parts of the world the medications may be sold under different trade names, so when traveling, take a list of the chemical names, or generic names, of the drugs you are taking:

Apokyn is apomorphine
Artane is trihexyphenidyl
Azilect is rasagiline
Cogentin is benztropine
Comtan is entacapone
Eldepryl is selegiline
Mirapex is pramipexole (also available in long-acting form)
Parcopa is carbidopa/levodopa
Parlodel is bromocriptine
Permax is pergolide
Requip is ropinirole (also available in long-acting form)
Sinemet is carbidopa/levodopa
Sinemet CR is carbidopa/levodopa
Stalevo is carbidopa/levodopa/entacapone
Neuropro is rotigotine
Symmetrel is amantadine
Tasmar is tolcapone
Zydis Selegiline is selegiline

(See Chapter 13 for the generic names of other drugs you may be taking that are not listed here.) If you run out of medication or need advice about your medicine while on vacation, you can tell the local doctor or pharmacist the chemical name of the drug, and the doctor or pharmacist should be able to supply the equivalent medication.

Q: Is there any problem in transporting my medication across national borders?

A: You should not have any difficulty in carrying the medications you need for your own health across national borders. It might be beneficial to have a note from your doctor indicating that you take these drugs, in case any questions arise from border officials. If you are traveling for a long period and are carrying a large quantity of medication in your suitcase, customs or drug enforcement officials may be suspicious. A letter from your doctor or pharmacist stating the name of the drug, the number of pills you take each day, and the quantity of pills you require for a long trip might prove useful in these circumstances.

Q: When traveling, do I need a letter from my doctor explaining my medication?

A: A list of the medications you are taking, with their generic or chemical names, will prove useful if you require medical attention.

MEDICATIONS

Q: Are there interactions between antiparkinson medications and common over-the-counter medications such as analgesics, cold remedies and anti-inflammatory drugs, or prescription medications such as antibiotics, sleeping pills, antidepressants, and anxiolytics?

A: The drugs used to treat Parkinson's disease are remarkably free of drug interactions. People taking carbidopa/levodopa (Sinemet or Sinemet CR), dopamine agonists (including Apokyn, Mirapex, Requip, Permax, and Parlodel or the Rotigotine patch), anticholinergics (including Artane, Kemadrin, Parsitan, and Cogentin), amantadine (Symmetrel), or MAO-B inhibitors (including rasagiline and selegiline) can take Tylenol (acetaminophen), aspirin, or other anti-inflammatory drugs such as Motrin (ibuprofen) and Advil (ibuprofen) without any fear of interaction. Antibiotics, when necessary to treat infectious processes, can also be taken without interfering with the antiparkinson drugs. Medications taken to treat anxiety (the so-called minor tranquilizers, including Valium, Tranxene, Ativan, and Xanax) and most antidepressants can also be used (in proper dosages, of course) without fear of interaction with the antiparkinson drugs. Antihistamines and other over-the-counter cold remedies (upper respiratory treatment) can also be safely taken with antiparkinson's disease drugs. In recent years, there has been quite a bit of confusion among patients and families, because there are warnings on these cold remedies stating not to take them if using antiparkinson's disease drugs. We have never encountered any problems in our patients when cold remedies and Parkinson's disease medication are used together, and we routinely advise patients that this combination is safe.

Q: What drugs should be avoided by someone with Parkinson's disease?

A: People who have Parkinson's should avoid strong psychiatric medications known as neuroleptics and major tranquilizers, including thioridazine (Mellaril), haloperidol (Haldol), trifluoperazine (Stelazine), chlorpromazine (Thorazine), and perphenazine (Trilafon), which are used to treat psychosis and schizophrenia. These drugs block the effect of dopamine and disrupt the effects of the antiparkinson drugs. Metoclopramide (Reglan), commonly used to treat gastrointestinal disorders, and prochlorperazine (Compazine), used to treat nausea, should also be avoided, because they also interfere with the action of antiparkinson drugs. Blood pressure medication containing reserpine should not be used. All these medications will make the symptoms of Parkinson's disease worse. A new class of tranquilizing drugs called "atypical" antipsychotics can also interfere with dopamine activity in the brain. In particular, risperidone (Risperdal) and olanzapene (Zyprexa) should be avoided. There is less experience with aripiprazole (Abilify), and ziprasidone (Geodon), but it does seem that these medications can also cause an increase in parkinsonism. Quetiapine (Seroquel) is less likely to interfere with dopamine activity in the brain, but its efficacy for psychotic symptoms in Parkinson's disease is quite variable. The safest (with respect to aggravating motor symptoms of parkinsonism) and most effective antipsychotic drug for people who have Parkinson's disease is clozapine, but taking this drug requires the patient to have regular blood monitoring (see Chapter 13).

Q: When should antiparkinson medication be started?

A: At the present time, all antiparkinson medications simply improve the symptoms of Parkinson's disease without altering the course of the disease. For this reason, a person who has Parkinson's usually doesn't begin taking medications until she or he begins to experience some degree of disability. This may occur when tremor becomes pronounced and troublesome, or when dexterity is compromised, or when work or a favorite recreational activity is threatened (Chapter 12). These are all appropriate reasons to begin medication.

Of course, if drugs are eventually developed that can suppress or slow the disease process, it will become very important to start medication as soon as the diagnosis is made. At the present time, drugs of this nature simply do not exist, and so physicians must be guided by the symptomatic needs of their patients.

Q: Is it true that levodopa preparations such as Sinemet, Sinemet CR, Prolopa, and Madopar only work for a limited period of time?

A: No. Levodopa is the most potent medication to treat the symptoms of Parkinson's disease, and it remains effective throughout the course of the illness. Levodopa continues to maintain its effectiveness for Parkinson's symptoms despite prolonged use. What happens, however, is that as the symptoms become more advanced and severe, they can no longer be fully relieved throughout the day. In this sense, the action of levodopa can be compared to the action of a pain medication that completely eliminates a moderate headache but only "dulls" the pain of a severe headache (Chapter 13)—it's not that the pain medication doesn't "work," but the pain is too severe to be controlled by the pain medication. Some symptoms, for example tremor and rigidity, can continue to respond equally well to levodopa after ten to twenty years (or more) of treatment as they did at the onset of therapy. Others, such as speech difficulties, walking problems, unsteadiness, and the tendency to fall, become increasingly resistant to levodopa over the years. One explanation for this resistance is that these symptoms are due to degeneration of brain regions other than the substantia nigra and are therefore not caused by dopamine deficiency. Treatment of these late-stage "nondopaminergic" symptoms is one of the most important challenges in the modern therapy of Parkinson's disease.

Patients sometimes think they should delay treatment until later in the disease, when they will "really need it," since they think that the medications will only help for a finite time. However, as indicated above, this is simply incorrect. Delaying levodopa in the early years of the disease can result in the person unnecessarily experiencing disability that can have a negative impact on their enjoyment of life, including social and family interactions. In addition, delaying levodopa does not translate into the drug being more effective later in the disease, since it will help the dopamine-related symptoms both early and late but will not improve the nondopamine-related symptoms that become more of a problem later in the disease.

Q: Do levodopa and other medications cause abnormal involuntary movements and hallucinations?

A: The abnormal movements that appear with long-term use of carbidopa/levodopa and dopamine agonists are called dyskinesia. Although not everyone with Parkinson's disease will develop dyskinesia, it is very common after five to ten years of levodopa therapy. The movements can be controlled by changing the dose and timing of the antiparkinson medications. In 20 to 30 percent of people taking levodopa and dopamine receptor agonists, some psychiatric side effects develop, which include vivid dreams, benign or nonthreatening transient visual hallucinations, paranoia, and even overt psychotic behavior. These side effects, too, can be controlled by altering the antiparkinson medications as well as by taking so-called atypical antipsychotic medications such as clozapine (Clozaril) or quetiapine (Seroquel) (Chapter 13).

Q: Can vitamin E help people who have Parkinson's disease?

A: After careful study, investigators have concluded that vitamin E (tocopherol), even in dosages as large as 2,000 units a day, does not slow the progression of the disease; nor does it have any beneficial effect on the symptoms of Parkinson's disease (Chapter 15). Some people believe higher dosages of vitamin E may be required to show any effect, but dosages higher than 2,000 units a day may cause adverse effects.

Q: Can vitamin C help?

A: A few small, uncontrolled clinical studies have suggested that vitamin C might slow the progression of Parkinson's disease, but the current evidence is very weak. There is no widespread acceptance of the idea that vitamin C alters Parkinson's disease in any way. The dosage of vitamin C that has been recommended for Parkinson's is 2 to 3 grams a day, but, again, we have no evidence to support its use. Most movement disorder specialists do not recommend that their patients take high-dose vitamin C in the course of their illness (Chapter 15).

Q: What about vitamin B_6?

A: Many people who have Parkinson's disease believe that ingesting vitamin B_6 (pyridoxine) is detrimental. This belief stems from what is now a historical period in the treatment of Parkinson's disease, when levodopa was administered alone, without a peripheral dopamine decarboxylase inhibitor such as carbidopa. When levodopa was used alone, vitamin B_6 interfered with the transport of dopamine into the brain (Chapter 15). But vitamin B_6 can be taken by people who use carbidopa/levodopa, without any detrimental effects. The vitamin B_6 found in multivitamins and in cereals or other foods does not interfere with the effectiveness of Sinemet or Sinemet CR (or Madopar and Prolopa, in other countries).

Q: Should I take Coenzyme Q_{10} (CoQ_{10})?

A: Coenzyme Q_{10} is a nutritional supplement that is being investigated to see whether or not it can slow disease progression in Parkinson's disease. In a well-conducted earlier trial, there was a suggestion that 1,200 milligrams of CoQ_{10} a day might be helpful, while doses smaller than 1,200 milligrams a day were not effective. In the much larger trial of CoQ_{10} in early Parkinson's disease, 2,400 mg/day was used to investigate the concept that CoQ10 might slow progression of Parkinson's disease. Unfortunately, this trial, sponsored by the NIH, was stopped because the high dose did not slow Parkinson's disease progression. Your insurance company will not pay for CoQ_{10} because it is not considered a drug. We advise our patients that taking this supplement for neuroprotection has no proven value. Importantly, most forms of CoQ_{10} available in health food stores contain much smaller amounts of the coenzyme than were studied, and many products may not even contain the amount they claim. Keep in mind that health foods (which include nutritional supplements) are not regulated for content in the same way pharmaceuticals are.

Q: How should I time my medication around meals?
A: The only medication that may be affected by meals is carbidopa/ levodopa (and other levodopa preparations), which is more effective if taken twenty to thirty minutes *before* eating. However, taking carbidopa/levodopa on an empty stomach is more likely to cause gastrointestinal upset such as nausea and vomiting, in which case the medication must be taken with a meal. Eating a high-protein meal with, or soon after taking, a dose of carbidopa/levodopa may decrease the effectiveness of the medication in some people, and these people may do better by following the protein redistribution diet (Chapters 13 and 15). Dopamine receptor agonists (Parlodel, NeuproMirapex, and Requip), tolcapone (Tasmar), entacapone (Comtan), selegiline (Eldepryl), rasagiline (Azilect), anticholinergics (Artane, Kemadrin, and Cogentin), and amantadine (Symmetrel) can be taken before, during, or after a meal without any concern about altering their effectiveness.

Q: How critical is it that I take my medication at specific times?
A: You should take medication for Parkinson's disease on a regular schedule so your body can become accustomed to a routine schedule of doses, rather than having to cope with erratic dosing. Following a medication schedule is also extremely important to help your physician do the best possible job in managing your symptoms. Fine-tuning of the control of Parkinson's symptoms requires a reliable medication history as well as reliable reporting of symptoms. The importance of staying on schedule increases as the symptoms of Parkinson's disease progress. Early in the illness the symptoms are "forgiving," and medication can be taken early or late without sacrificing control of symptoms. As the symptoms become more advanced, a delay of even fifteen or thirty minutes can substantially affect a person's ability to function.

Q: What should I do if I forget to take a dose of medication?
A: If you do not experience motor fluctuations and you forget to take a dose of medication, you probably won't feel the consequences

of missing just a single dose. There is no need to make up the dose or double-up on the next dose. But if you have more advanced disease and you experience "wearing-off" of the drug's effectiveness with motor fluctuations, the delay in taking medication will likely result in increased disability due to more "off" time. When this is the case, you will probably need to add the missed dose back into your schedule. The dose should be taken immediately, and you may then need to adjust the timing of the remaining daily doses accordingly.

Disability

Q: Will I eventually require live-in help?
A: Parkinson's disease is a progressive illness, but in each person the disease progresses at a different rate. Not everyone with Parkinson's eventually requires live-in help, but many people eventually do become sufficiently disabled that they require help (at least at some time during the day) with many household functions.

Q: Will I ever require nursing home care?
A: Some people who have Parkinson's disease eventually become so disabled that they have to be cared for in a nursing home. On the other hand, many people who have Parkinson's never require nursing home care. In addition to the central issue of disease severity and disability, other important issues determine whether an individual requires care in a nursing home: the level of family support available, the person's and the family's financial situation, and the degree of cognitive impairment. Adequate financial resources and family support may enable a person to remain at home.

Q: As my disease progresses, will I be able to control my bladder and bowels?
A: Bladder and bowel problems are common in advanced Parkinson's disease (Chapter 5), but urinary and bowel incontinence are extremely rare. When bladder and bowel problems occur early in the course of a person's illness, it is likely that she or he does not have true Parkinson's disease, but rather a related Parkinson's-plus syndrome (Chapter 10).

Q: Is there sex after Parkinson's disease?

A: The continuation of a healthy sexual relationship is especially important to a person who has a chronic neurologic disorder. In early, mild Parkinson's disease, people seldom have problems with erection and orgasm, but there may be psychological issues such as concerns about body image, feeling less sexually desirable, depression, and anxiety. As physical disability increases, physical mobility and dexterity become more of an issue. Sexual partners need to be good communicators to compensate for these changes.

Men with Parkinson's disease may experience erectile dysfunction (impotence), which sometimes occurs relatively early in the illness. There are a number of ways of treating this problem, including the oral medications sildenafil (Viagra), vardenafil (Levitra), and tadalafil (Cialis), and medications that are administered by injection directly into the penis (Chapter 5). Very little information is available on the sexual experience or the proper treatment of sexual difficulties of women with Parkinson's. Medical diagnostic investigations, psychological counseling, and a variety of therapeutic interventions can be helpful. Some people, most often men, experience an increase in sexual drive in response to certain antiparkinson medications, and at times this can reach a level that creates important problems in the patient's marital relationship. This, too, should be brought to the attention of the doctor, as medication adjustments may be necessary.

Q: Will Parkinson's disease shorten my life? Is it fatal?

A: Parkinson's disease is not a fatal illness. It is a chronic, progressive disease that results in many areas of disability. The disability and immobility related to Parkinson's can result in life-threatening illnesses, such as aspiration pneumonia or urinary tract infection (Chapter 5). The care of people who have advanced disease involves vigilance and prevention to protect them from complications that can place them at risk. Parkinson's disease alone does not significantly affect longevity.

Q: What is a drug holiday?

A: *Drug holiday* is a term that was applied to a particular therapy in patients with Parkinson's disease that is now rarely used. A *drug holiday* consisted of withdrawing all levodopa from a patient with Parkinson's disease who was not doing well. The withdrawal of all levodopa resulted in marked worsening of all symptoms and the theory was that improvement might be obtained for the patient when levodopa was restarted (a form of resensitization to the drug). Unfortunately, the improvement was only short lived and the complications were quite dramatic, including marked and severe worsening of motor abilities, deep vein thrombosis (blood clots in the legs), swallowing difficulties, and aspiration pneumonia. When it is necessary to make a dramatic change in Parkinson's medication it should be done under the supervision of an experienced neurologist.

Q: What is the role of exercise in the management of Parkinson's disease?

A: Exercise programs play a significant role in the treatment of Parkinson's disease. How to exercise (the type of exercise), how often, and how vigorously have not yet been determined, but it appears from recent studies that both intensity and duration of exercise are important (see Chapter 14).

Q: When is the "stem cell cure" going to be available?

A: There has been a great deal of publicity surrounding the potential for stem cells to cure Parkinson's disease. Indeed, it was once widely believed that Parkinson's disease was the "poster-child for stem cell research," because it was thought that stem cells could provide an infinite supply of dopamine cells that could be implanted into the brain of people who have Parkinson's—replacing degenerating cells of the substantia nigra. However, there are many problems with this simplistic concept. First, we know from the fetal transplant experience (Chapter 16) that many patients do not seem to benefit from replacing dopamine cells into the brain. Second, again from the fetal transplant experience, transplant-induced dyskinesias are a problem that could also occur with dopamine cells arising from stem cells. Third, as has been repeatedly emphasized in this book, Parkinson's disease is recognized as being more than a pure dopamine deficiency state, and the nondopamine features remain some of the most disabling features, especially later in the disease. Using stem cells to fix the dopamine deficiency would not be expected to have any impact on these features.

Since the nondopamine features relate to dysfunction of many diverse brain cell types and brain regions, a great deal more research will be needed before we might understand how stems cells could overcome these problems. In some countries, such as China and some Eastern European countries (and until recently Germany), stem cell treatment is offered through injections into cerebrospinal fluid in the spinal canal (intrathecal injections). The origin of these cells is often unclear to those not involved in the procedure (sometimes they are taken from the patient's bone marrow), and there is no evidence whatsoever that this treatment influences the disease beyond a placebo effect, that the cells even survive, or that the treatment is truly safe. We feel that centers offering this treatment now are making completely unfounded claims and are preying on patients' hopes and on their frustrations with the limitations of our current therapy. We very strongly recommend against patients receiving these treatments.

On the other hand, advances in credible stem cell research may eventually have a significant impact on our understanding of Parkinson's disease and its treatment. We simply need to have a realistic view of what is possible now and a hope that future research will make some of the past expectations a reality.

Q: Does my spouse have Lewy body disease instead of Parkinson's?
A: This is a common question arising when families dealing with dementia-complicating later-stage Parkinson's disease read about Dementia with Lewy Bodies (DLB) or they see another physician who suggests this "new" diagnosis. As discussed in Chapter 10, it is generally believed that Parkinson's disease dementia (PDD) and DLB are very similar if not identical when the brains are studied at autopsy. The time of onset of dementia is the differentiating feature: the first symptom (or in the first year) in DLB and after one or typically many years of Parkinson's symptoms in PDD.

Resources

American Academy of Neurology (AAN), 201 Chicago Avenue South, Minneapolis, MN 55415. Toll-free number: 1-800-879-1960. Or call 612-928-6000. Web site: www.aan.com.

The American Academy of Neurology is the world's largest association of neurologists with 24,000 members dedicated to promoting the highest quality patient-centered neurologic care for people including those living with Parkinson's disease. Free resources for these patients and their caregivers include the Academy's award-winning magazine *Neurology Now* and its Web site www.aan.com/patients, which includes the latest information on Parkinson's disease, as well as videos, patient stories, and a Find a Neurologist Tool to locate a neurologist near you who treats Parkinson's disease. Patients may also call the Academy at 1-800-879-1960 for more information.

American Parkinson Disease Association, Inc. (APDA), 135 Parkinson Avenue, Staten Island, NY 10305. Toll-free number: 1-800-223-2732. Web site: www.apdaparkinson.org.

American Parkinson Disease Association, Inc. (APDA), operating through a national network of volunteer chapters, professionally staffed information and referral centers, and more than a thousand support groups, is the largest grassroots organization serving America's 1.5 million people who have Parkinson's disease. It is a nonprofit organization that sponsors a comprehensive program of research, patient education, and support, including the only national center for young-onset patients and their families, and the only national resource center for rehabilitation. APDA currently funds nine centers for advanced research. The organization publishes numerous booklets and educational supplements, a quarterly newsletter, a monthly e-newsletter and "Tip of the Month" service, maintains two national Web sites (www.apdaparkinson.org and www.youngparkinsons.org), and provides a free online private caregiver coordination service.

The Michael J. Fox Foundation for Parkinson's Research, Grand Central Station, P.O. Box 4777, New York, NY 10163. Toll-free number: 1-800-708-7644. Web site: www.michaeljfox.org.

Established in 2000, the Michael J. Fox Foundation for Parkinson's Research seeks to identify the most promising research into a cure for Parkinson's and to raise the necessary funds to ensure that such research is supported. Since its inception in 2000, the Foundation has funded over $120 million in both basic and clinical research in Parkinson's disease.

Movement Disorder Society. Web site: www.movementdisorders.org.

National Institute of Neurological Disorders and Stroke (NINDS), P.O. Box 5801, Bethesda, MD 20824. Toll-free number: 1-800-532-9424. Web site: www.ninds.nih.gov.

Part of the National Institutes of Health, NINDS conducts and coordinates research on the causes, prevention, and treatment of neurologic disorders and strokes, including Parkinson's disease. NINDS also collects and disseminates research information on neurologic disorders. Updates on the NINDS's research agenda for Parkinson's disease can be found on its Web site: www.ninds.nih.gov/news_and_events/index.htm.

The National Parkinson Foundation, Inc. (NPF), 1501 N.W. 9th Avenue, Bob Hope Road, Miami, FL 33136. Toll-free number: 1-800-327-4545. Web site: www.parkinson.org. Email: contact@parkinson.org.

Founded in 1961, the NPF is a nonprofit organization devoted to finding the cause of and discovering the cure for Parkinson's disease. In addition to conducting research at its headquarters at the University of Miami's Departments of Neurology and Neurosurgery, the NPF sponsors research at more than fifty centers located in the United States and other countries. The NPF has a toll-free number for patients' questions and physician referrals, as well as an interactive Web site. The NPF has a quarterly publication, *Parkinson Report,* and provides other materials on Parkinson's disease treatment and research free of charge to patients, physicians, and researchers.

Parkinson Society Canada, 4211 Yonge Street, Suite 316, Toronto, Ontario M2P 2A9, Canada. Toll-free number: 1-800-565-3000. Web site: www.par kinson.ca.

Parkinson Society Canada (PSC) is a national nonprofit charity supporting Canadians touched by Parkinson's since 1965. PSC funds a national research program, provides education and support to ensure a better quality of life, and advocates for better policies. In partnership with ten regional offices and over 240 chapters and support groups across Canada, PSC provides information and referrals to community resources in both English and French via a toll-free telephone service. PSC produces informational materials including fact sheets, handbooks, an electronic newsletter, e-Parkisonpost, and an annual Research Highlights publication. Parkinson Society Canada was instrumental in initiating the first Canadian Guidelines on Parkinson's Disease (June 2012). To learn more, visit www.parkinson.ca.

Parkinson Study Group (PSG), University of Rochester, 1351 Mount Hope Avenue, Suite 223, Rochester, NY 14620. Telephone: 716-275-1935. Web site: www.parkinson-study-group.org.

Founded in 1986, the PSG is a nonprofit group of physicians and other health care professionals who are experienced in the care of people who have Parkinson's and dedicated to research on Parkinson's disease. The consortium consists of more than 233 investigators, coordinators, and consulting scientists from more than fifty participating sites in the United States and Canada. Since its founding, the PSG has conducted twenty-five multicenter controlled clinical trials to study new treatments for Parkinson's disease. The PSG seeks to foster open communication within the scientific community and to ensure that the results of Parkinson's research are available to the public. The PSG regularly reports the findings of its studies at national and international medical meetings and in medical journals.

Parkinson's Action Network, 1025 Vermont Avenue, N.W., Suite 1120, Washington, DC 20005. Toll-free number: 1-800-850-4726. Web site: www.parkinsonsaction.org. Email: info@parkinsonsaction.org.

The Parkinson's Action Network (PAN) is the unified voice of the Parkinson's community advocating for better treatments and a cure. In partnership with other Parkinson's organizations and the network's powerful grassroots network, PAN educates the public and government leaders on better policies for research and an improved quality of life for people living with Parkinson's.

Parkinson's Disease Foundation, Inc., 1359 Broadway, Suite 1509, New York, NY 10018. Toll-free number: 1-800-457-6676. Web site: www.pdf.org. Email: info@pdf.org.

The Parkinson's Disease Foundation (PDF) funds research and leads innovative national education and advocacy initiatives that seek to improve the lives and futures of people touched by Parkinson's disease. PDF's educational programs include a toll-free HelpLine, which provides information about Parkinson's and referrals to local support groups and resources; bimonthly online seminars led by Parkinson's experts; and free print publications. PDF also offers online courses and resources for health care professionals, including nurses and physical therapists. PDF's primary advocacy program, Parkinson's Advocates in Research, trains people who have Parkinson's and care partners to influence research and speed new and effective treatments for Parkinson's.

WE MOVE (Worldwide Education and Awareness for Movement Disorders), 204 West 84th Street, New York, NY 10024. Toll-free number: 1-800-437-MOV2. Web site: www.wemove.org. Email: wemove@wemove.org.

WE MOVE is a nonprofit organization that works to educate health care professionals, patients, and the public about movement disorders, including Parkinson's disease. The organization offers several resources for medical professionals, including online educational programs, office resources including handouts for patients, and a research news service. WE MOVE also provides resources for patients and their families, including information on disorders and treatment, news on the latest research, discussion forums and webinars, and a schedule of regional and national support group events.

World Parkinson Disease Association (WPDA), via Zuretti, 35, 20125 Milan, Italy. Telephone: 39-02-66713111. Web site: www.wpda.org. Email: info@ wpda.org.

Established in 1998, the WPDA is a nonprofit organization that seeks to improve the quality of life of Parkinson's patients throughout the world through education and to foster improved communication and cooperation among patients' organizations from different countries. The Association also encourages the standardization of diagnostic procedures as well as medical and surgical therapies. In addition to supporting research on Parkinson's disease, the WPDA offers educational materials to patients both online and in print. Although based in Italy, the official language of the WPDA is English.

Index

Italic page number refer to figures; "t" refers to tables.